HPNA PALLIATIVE NURSING MANUALS

Care of the Imminently Dying

HPNA PALLIATIVE NURSING MANUALS

Series edited by: Betty R. Ferrell, RN, PhD, MA, FAAN, FPCN, CHPN

Volume 1: Structure and Processes of Care

Volume 2: Physical Aspects of Care: Pain and Gastrointestinal Symptoms

Volume 3: Physical Aspects of Care: Nutritional, Dermatologic, Neurologic, and Other Symptoms

Volume 4: Pediatric Palliative Care

Volume 5: Spiritual, Religious, and Cultural Aspects of Care

Volume 6: Social Aspects of Care

Volume 7: Care of the Imminently Dying

Volume 8: Ethical and Legal Aspects of Care

HPNA PALLIATIVE NURSING MANUALS

Care of the Imminently Dying

Edited by

Judith A. Paice, PhD, RN, FAAN

Director of Cancer Pain Program
Feinberg School of Medicine
Northwestern University
Chicago, Illinois

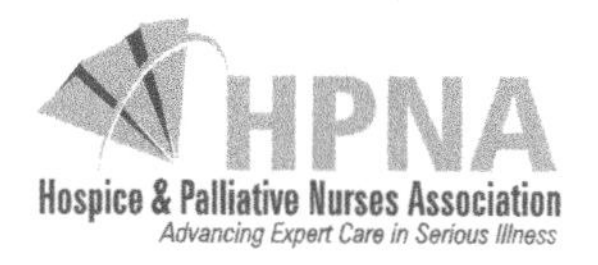

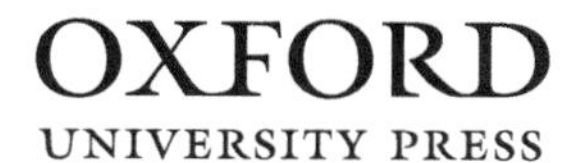

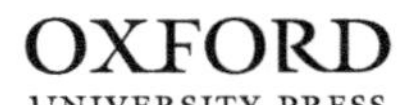

Oxford University Press is a department of the University of Oxford. It furthers the University's objective of excellence in research, scholarship, and education by publishing worldwide.

Oxford New York
Auckland Cape Town Dar es Salaam Hong Kong Karachi
Kuala Lumpur Madrid Melbourne Mexico City Nairobi
New Delhi Shanghai Taipei Toronto

With offices in
Argentina Austria Brazil Chile Czech Republic France Greece
Guatemala Hungary Italy Japan Poland Portugal Singapore
South Korea Switzerland Thailand Turkey Ukraine Vietnam

Oxford is a registered trademark of Oxford University Press
in the UK and certain other countries.

Published in the United States of America by
Oxford University Press
198 Madison Avenue, New York, NY 10016

© Oxford University Press 2016

All rights reserved. No part of this publication may be reproduced, stored in a retrieval system, or transmitted, in any form or by any means, without the prior permission in writing of Oxford University Press, or as expressly permitted by law, by license, or under terms agreed with the appropriate reproduction rights organization. Inquiries concerning reproduction outside the scope of the above should be sent to the Rights Department, Oxford University Press, at the address above.

You must not circulate this work in any other form
and you must impose this same condition on any acquirer.

Library of Congress Cataloging-in-Publication Data
Care of the imminently dying / edited by Judith A. Paice.
p. ; cm. — (HPNA palliative nursing manuals; v. 7)
Includes bibliographical references.
ISBN 978–0–19–024428–6 (alk. paper)
I. Paice, Judith A., editor. II. Series: HPNA palliative nursing manuals ; v. 7.
[DNLM: 1. Hospice and Palliative Care Nursing—methods. 2. Chronic Disease—nursing. 3. Palliative Care—methods. 4. Terminal Care—methods. WY 152.3]
RT87.T45
616.02′9—dc23
2015023115

This material is not intended to be, and should not be considered, a substitute for medical or other professional advice. Treatment for the conditions described in this material is highly dependent on the individual circumstances. And, while this material is designed to offer accurate information with respect to the subject matter covered and to be current as of the time it was written, research and knowledge about medical and health issues are constantly evolving, and dose schedules for medications are being revised continually, with new side effects recognized and accounted for regularly. Readers must therefore always check the product information and clinical procedures with the most up-to-date published product information and data sheets provided by the manufacturers and the most recent codes of conduct and safety regulations. The publisher and the authors make no representations or warranties to readers, express or implied, as to the accuracy or completeness of this material. Without limiting the foregoing, the publisher and the authors make no representations or warranties as to the accuracy or efficacy of the drug dosages mentioned in the material. The authors and the publisher do not accept, and expressly disclaim, any responsibility for any liability, loss, or risk that may be claimed or incurred as a consequence of the use and/or application of any of the contents of this material.

9 8 7 6 5 4 3 2
Printed in Canada
on acid-free paper

Contents

Preface

This is the seventh volume of a new series being published by Oxford University Press in collaboration with the Hospice and Palliative Nurses Association. The intent of this series is to provide palliative care nurses with quick reference guides to each of the key domains of palliative care.

Content for this series was derived primarily from the *Oxford Textbook of Palliative Nursing* (4th edition, 2015), which is also edited by Betty Ferrell, Nessa Coyle, and Judith Paice, the editors of this series. The contributors identified in each volume are the authors of chapters in the *Oxford Textbook of Palliative Nursing* from which the content was selected for this volume. The *Textbook* contains more extensive content and references, so users of this Palliative Nursing Series are encouraged to use the *Textbook* as an additional resource.

We are grateful to all palliative care nurses who are contributing to the advancement of care for seriously ill patients and families. Remarkable progress has occurred over the past 30 years in this field, and nurses have been central to that progress. Our hope is that this series offers an additional tool to build the care delivery system we strive for.

Contributors

Barton T. Bobb, MSN, FNP-BC, ACHPN
Palliative Care and Pain Consult Team
VCU Medical Center
Richmond, Virginia

Margaret L. Campbell, PhD, RN, FPCN
Professor of Research
College of Nursing
Wayne State University
Detroit, Michigan

Deborah Dudgeon, MD, FRCPC
W. Ford Connell Professor of Palliative Care Medicine
Department of Medicine
Oncology and Family Medicine
Queen's University
Kingston, Ontario, Canada

Nancy K. English, PhD, APRN, CN, CHPN
Adjunct Assistant Professor of Nursing
University of Colorado Health Sciences
Aurora, Colorado

Laura A. Espinosa, RN, MS, PhD
Instructor
The Methodist Hospital Research Institute
Director of Nursing
Methodist West Houston Hospital
Houston, Texas

Bonnie Freeman, RN, MSN, ANP-BC, CHPN
Supportive Care Medicine
Pain and Palliative Care Medicine
City of Hope National Medical Center
Duarte, California

Linda M. Gorman, RN, MN, PMHCNS-BC, CHPN, OCN, FPCN
Palliative Care Clinical Nurse Specialist and Consultant
Los Angeles, California

Debra E. Heidrich, MSN, RN, ACHPN, AOCN
Palliative Care Clinical Nurse Specialist
Bethesda North Hospital, TriHealth, Inc.
Cincinnati, Ohio

Patti Knight, RN, MSN, CS, CHPN
Palliative Care Unit Patient Manager
Department of Palliative Care and Rehabilitation Medicine
University of Texas M. D. Anderson Cancer Center
Houston, Texas

Chapter 1

Delirium

Debra E. Heidrich and Nancy K. English

Introduction

Delirium is a common neuropsychiatric disorder seen in all healthcare settings and is frequently underdiagnosed, misdiagnosed, and poorly managed. Often, patients are labeled as "confused," and no further evaluation is performed to determine the cause of this confusion. This is particularly an issue with elderly patients, whose confusion is often dismissed as dementia, and for those with terminal illness, whose confusion may be accepted as part of disease progression. Patients at highest risk for delirium include those who are elderly, in intensive care units, or postoperative as well as those with advanced illnesses. This syndrome is associated with significant morbidity and mortality, leading to increased length of hospital and nursing home stays and risk for earlier death. The experience of delirium is frightening to both patients and their significant others; it impairs quality of living—and quality of dying. Prompt recognition and treatment are essential to improve patient outcomes, especially in the final stages of an illness.

Incidence, Prevalence, and Outcomes

Delirium is considered the most common and serious cognitive disorder in hospitals and in the palliative care setting.[1] Reported incidence and prevalence rates vary depending on the population being studied, criteria used to identify delirium, and setting. Delirium is reported to be found in 0.5% to 10% of community-based elders, 8.9% to 47% of institutionalized elders, 14% to 56% of hospitalized elders, 45% of elders after general anesthesia, 60% to 80% of mechanically ventilated adult patients in intensive care units, 26% to 62% of palliative care admissions, and 58.8% to 88% of persons in the weeks or hours preceding death.[2] However, the true incidence of delirium is unknown because it often goes undetected or misdiagnosed. Factors that contribute to a missed diagnosis include the following:

- History of a past psychiatric diagnosis or cognitive disorder, such as dementia, to which the symptoms may be attributed
- Acceptance of confusion as an expected consequence of old age and dying
- Presence of pain
- Transient and fluctuating nature of symptoms

- Imprecise and overlapping use of terminology, such as delirium, acute confusion, and terminal restlessness
- Inconsistencies in use of and types of assessment tools used to diagnose delirium

Delirium is associated with adverse physical, cognitive, and psychological outcomes. It is associated with short- and long-term decline in cognitive functioning and increases in falls, length of hospital stays, need for institutionalized care after hospitalization, and mortality. Although not everyone remembers their experience of delirium, those who do remember report having distressing feelings during the experience, including fear, anxiety, and feeling threatened.[3]

- Visual hallucinations of people or animals in the room intertwine with the people who are actually present to create a confusing and frightening experience.
- Procedures like injections may be interpreted as attempts to do harm, and interventions to reorient or reassure delirious patients may be met with suspicion and the fear that everyone is lying to them.
- Feeling threatened, the delirious patient may try to escape from the experience, leading to wandering behavior and falls as well as aggression toward caregivers.
- After the episode of delirium, persons report feeling humiliated and ashamed of their behavior while delirious. They also report a fear of experiencing delirium again in the future and may exhibit signs of post-traumatic stress disorder.
- Caregivers also experience distress related to delirium. Family members recall more symptoms of delirium than both the patient and the bedside nurse and are more distressed by the experience. Agitation and delusions or hallucinations are particularly distressing to both family members and nurses.
- Interventions to decrease the incidence of delirium and prompt treatment of delirium symptoms may help decrease caregiver distress.
- Providing information about delirium and support throughout this difficult time may reduce both acute and long-term distress in family members.[3]

Restlessness or agitation at the end of life, sometimes called "terminal restlessness" or "terminal delirium," has been viewed as an expected part of the dying process.[4] However, descriptions of terminal restlessness overlap considerably with the defining characteristics of delirium. Importantly, delirium is potentially reversible in some persons, even at the end of life. Given this potential for reversibility, a thorough evaluation of treatable causes of delirium is required, followed by appropriate interventions based on the patient's overall condition and the goals of care.

A comprehensive plan for delirium that includes prevention, assessment and early detection, and appropriate intervention has the potential to save lives, improve quality of life, and significantly decrease costs.

Definition and Key Features of Delirium

Understanding the many symptoms, syndromes, and diagnoses associated with cognitive changes in persons with an advanced illness can be difficult at best. Terms such as confusion, acute confusion, delirium, and terminal restlessness are often used to describe changes in mental status without clear definitions or use of standard psychiatric classifications. The use of imprecise terminology can lead to mislabeling of behaviors, miscommunication among healthcare professionals, and misdiagnoses of cognitive changes. Therefore, the potential for the mismanagement of any cognitive change is extremely high.

The fifth edition of the *Diagnostic and Statistical Manual of Mental Disorders* (DSM-5) criteria for delirium are listed in Box 1.1.[5] Key features are that the disturbances develop over a short period of time, tend to fluctuate in severity during the course of a day, and represent a change from baseline. There are no diagnostic tests for delirium; the diagnosis is primarily clinical, based on careful observation and awareness of the criteria. Because the presentation of symptoms can sometimes be subtle, and symptoms fluctuate throughout the day, nurses, who have more frequent and continuous contact with patients, are crucial to the early recognition of delirium.

Disturbance in attention refers to a reduced ability to direct, focus, sustain, and shift attention. In delirium, the disturbed attention is combined with a *disturbance in awareness*, defined as having a reduced orientation to the environment. Patients may be hypoalert, slow to respond, or unable to maintain eye contact, or they may fall asleep between stimuli, requiring an increased amount of stimuli (touch, calling name) to elicit a response. Conversely, patients may be hyperalert, overreact to stimuli, startle easily, rapidly change from one topic to another in conversation, and exhibit signs of agitation. In the early stage of delirium, the abnormalities in attention and awareness may be subtle and easily overlooked.

Box 1.1 Diagnostic Criteria for Delirium

Disturbance in Attention and Awareness

The disturbance develops over a short period of time and tends to fluctuate in severity during the course of the day.

Disturbance in Cognition

The disturbances in criteria A and C are not explained by another preexisting, established, or evolving neurocognitive disorder; and do not occur in the context of a severely reduced level of arousal, such as coma.

History, physical examination, or laboratory findings indicate that the disturbance is caused by a medical condition, substance intoxication or withdrawal, or exposure to a toxin; or is because of multiple etiologies.

Source: Adapted from American Psychiatric Association. *Diagnostic and Statistical Manual of Mental Disorders (DSM-5)*. Arlington, VA: American Psychiatric Association; 2013.

Changes in cognition in delirium include memory deficit, disorientation, language disturbances, and perceptual disturbances. Disruptions in orientation usually manifest as disorientation to time or place, with time disorientation being the first to be affected. Short-term memory deficits are the most evident memory impairments. Patients may not remember conversations, television shows, or verbal instructions. Language disturbances include incoherent or jumbled speech, use of repetitive phrases, abnormally long pauses in the conversation, or difficulty finding the proper words to convey a message. Perceptual disturbances are no longer considered essential to the diagnosis of delirium.[1] When they are present, these disturbances may include misinterpretations, illusions, or hallucinations. Visual misperceptions and hallucinations are most common, but auditory, tactile, gustatory, and olfactory misperceptions or hallucinations can also occur.

Development over a short time and fluctuation during the course of the day are important considerations in both identifying delirium and differentiating it from dementia. In dementia, short-term memory problems occur progressively over months versus over hours or days with delirium. Importantly, persons with dementia are at high risk for developing delirium.[2] Obtaining a history of memory issues from the family is vital to establishing the patient's baseline because it is the change from the baseline that indicates delirium in persons with and without dementia.

Additional clinical features of delirium that are not included in the diagnostic criteria but are frequently present include sleep-wake cycle disruption, hallucinations or perceptual distortions, delusional or fixed false beliefs, and mood lability. Some of these features help in differentiating delirium from dementia because persons with dementia do not typically have delusions or hallucinations. "Sundowning," or increased confusion and agitation at night, should be viewed as a potential sign of delirium unless this behavior has been present for weeks to months in the person with dementia.

Subtypes of Delirium

There are three clinical subtypes of delirium based on arousal disturbance and psychomotor behavior: hyperactive, hypoactive, and mixed.

Hyperactive delirium is associated with hypervigilance, restlessness, and agitation.
Hypoactive delirium is characterized by confusion and somnolence.
The mixed subtype of delirium has alternating features of hyperactive and hypoactive delirium.

Subsyndromal delirium is described by some as occurring in persons who have some symptoms associated with delirium, but not enough symptoms to fit the criteria for the diagnosis of delirium. Persons who exhibit these more subtle symptoms are certainly at risk for developing the diagnosable syndrome of delirium. Clinicians need to intervene to eliminate as many factors that contribute to delirium as possible, and they need to monitor these patients routinely for progression to delirium.

Hyperactive delirium is identified more often in the clinical setting than the other subtypes because the symptoms of hypervigilence, restlessness, and agitation attract caregiver attention. However, the hypoactive and mixed forms appear to be more prevalent. The hypoactive form of delirium is likely underdiagnosed because symptoms are less noticeable, or it may be misdiagnosed as depression or fatigue.[2]

Delirium in the Final Days of Life and Death-Bed Phenomena

Most patients who exhibit signs of the dying process experience symptoms consistent with delirium.[4] In a retrospective review, Chirco, Dunn, and Robinson found that delirium usually occurs 24 to 48 hours before death, with subtle signs being evident approximately 7 days before death.[6] Delirium around the time of death is sometimes referred to as terminal restlessness, terminal delirium, terminal agitation, preterminal restlessness, preterminal delirium, or terminal psychosis. To avoid confusion, the qualifiers "terminal" and "preterminal" should be avoided, and standardized assessment tools should be used to diagnose delirium throughout the course of illness, including in the final phase of life.

Although delirium may be very frequent at the end of life, restless behaviors in the dying patient should not be accepted as simply "part of the dying process"; reversal of delirium maybe possible even in very advanced stages of illness.[4] An evaluation to determine reversibility of a delirium is essential to facilitate a conscious, comfortable death whenever possible.

As death draws near, patients may experience apparitions of "helpers" or family members who have died and now appear to the patient as "guides" in the transition from life to death. These have been called death-bed visions (DBVs), and these often bring comfort to both patient and family. Patients have reported seeing angels, religious figures, spiritual guides, and deceased loved ones. It has been reported that 10% of patients are aware and conscious before death. Of these, approximately 50% to 60% are reported to have experienced a DBV.[7]

Hospice nurses, Callanan and Kelly, refer to these kinds of phenomena as "nearing death awareness" and define this concept as a special knowledge about the process of dying that may reveal what dying is like or what is needed to die peacefully.[8] Themes of nearing death awareness include describing a place, talking to or being in the presence of someone who is not alive, knowing when death will occur, choosing the time of death, needing reconciliation, preparing for travel or change, being held back, and having symbolic dreams.

Death-bed phenomena may be differentiated from delirium-related hallucinations or misperceptions by observing verbal and nonverbal behaviors. Persons experiencing DBVs tend to be calm or questioning but not fearful of the visions, are able to focus their attention on the vision and describe the experience coherently to others, may converse with the persons in the vision, and are comforted and consoled by this experience.

Etiology

Delirium usually develops because of the interrelationship between patient vulnerability (predisposing factors) and noxious insults (precipitating factors).[9] Table 1.1 identifies some of the common predisposing and precipitating factors for delirium. Although a single precipitating factor in the predisposed

Table 1.1 Predisposing and Precipitating Factors for Delirium

Predisposing Factors	Precipitating Factors
Demographic characteristics	*Drugs*
Age of 65 years or older	Sedative hypnotics
Male sex	Narcotics
Cognitive status	Anticholinergic drugs
Dementia	Treatment with multiple drugs
Cognitive impairment	Alcohol or drug withdrawal
History of delirium	*Primary neurologic diseases*
Depression	Stroke, particularly nondominant hemispheric
Functional status	Intracranial bleeding
Functional dependence	Meningitis or encephalitis
Immobility	*Intercurrent illnesses*
Low level of activity	Infections
History of falls	Iatrogenic complications
Sensory impairment	Severe acute illness
Visual impairment	Hypoxia
Hearing impairment	Shock
Decreased oral intake	Fever or hypothermia
Dehydration	Anemia
Malnutrition	Dehydration
Drugs	Poor nutritional status
Treatment with multiple psychoactive drugs	Low serum albumin level
Treatment with many drugs	Metabolic derangements (e.g., electrolyte, glucose, acid–base)
Alcohol abuse	*Surgery*
Coexisting medical conditions	Orthopedic surgery
Severe illness	Cardiac surgery
Multiple coexisting conditions	Prolonged cardiopulmonary bypass
Chronic renal or hepatic disease	Noncardiac surgery
History of stroke	*Environmental*
Neurologic disease	Admission to an intensive care unit
Metabolic derangements	Use of physical restraints
Fracture or trauma	Use of bladder catheter
Terminal illness	Use of multiple procedures
Infection with human immunodeficiency virus	Pain
	Emotional stress
	Prolonged sleep deprivation

Source: Adapted from Inouye S. Delirium in older persons. *N Engl J Med*. 2006;354:1157–1165.

patient may be enough to lead to delirium (e.g., a single dose of an anticholinergic medication in a patient with dementia), there are often multiple factors involved in the development of delirium. Addressing only a single factor likely will not aid in improving delirium; an approach that addresses as many predisposing and precipitating factors as possible is needed for resolution.

Nurses must be aware of the increased risk for delirium in patients with dementia, carefully assess for signs of delirium, and work to eliminate or decrease precipitating factors that can be controlled. Too often, changes in behavior are dismissed as signs of the individual's dementia instead of being identified as signs of delirium. Table 1.2 identifies the factors that help in differentiating dementia from delirium.[10] Knowledge of the patient's baseline cognitive status is critical for identifying recent changes in cognition and attention.

Several studies have identified key factors that increase the risk for delirium in subsets of populations.

Despite an incidence rate of 40% to 80% in persons with cancer, delirium is rarely appreciated as a source of symptom distress in oncology settings.[11] Table 1.3 outlines the cancer-specific considerations as they relate to the risk factors for delirium, illustrating that persons with cancer have many predisposing risk factors and are exposed to multiple precipitating factors for delirium.

Studies of patients undergoing surgery showed that preoperative cognitive deficits, preexisting depression, and impaired vision are common predisposing factors for delirium; in addition, duration of surgery, prolonged intubation, surgery type, and elevated inflammatory markers are frequent precipitating factors for postoperative delirium.

In the hospice and palliative care setting, poor sleep quality, uncontrolled pain, multiple medications (including high dose opioids), dehydration, infection, dementia, and organ failure are associated with delirium.

Five risk factors for persistent delirium in elderly patients at discharge from the hospital include dementia, vision impairment, functional impairment, high comorbidity, and use of physical restraints during delirium.[9]

Assessment

Comprehensive and ongoing assessment is necessary to identify patients at risk for delirium and to enable early detection of delirium. Standardized assessment tools for delirium administered by healthcare providers trained in using these tools improves the identification of delirium in the clinical setting.[1] Assessment tools include those designed to screen for delirium symptoms, those designed to make a formal diagnosis of delirium, and those designed to rate the severity of delirium.

The Mini-Mental State Examination (MMSE) is a 20-item screening tool that provides a clinical evaluation of cognitive function but is not specifically designed to assess for delirium and does not differentiate between dementia and delirium.[12] It assesses orientation, attention, recall, and language function. The MMSE is widely used in practice and research, and data support the scoring system to identify the severity of cognitive impairment. The length of this

Table 1.2 Differentiating Delirium From Dementia

	Delirium	Dementia
Onset	Acute or subacute, occurs over a short period of time (hours to days).	Insidious, often slow and progressive.
Course	Fluctuates over the course of the day, worsens at night. Resolves over days to weeks.	Stable over the course of the day; is progressive.
Duration	If reversible, short term.	Chronic and nonreversible.
Consciousness	Impaired and can fluctuate rapidly. Clouded, with a reduced awareness of the environment.	Clear and alert until the later stages. May become delirious, which will interfere.
Cognitive defects	Impaired short-term memory, poor attention span.	Poor short-term memory; attention span less affected until later stage.
Attention	Reduced ability to focus, sustain, or shift attention.	Relatively unaffected in the earlier stages.
Orientation	Disoriented to time and place.	Intact until months or years with the later stages. May have anomia (difficulty recognizing common objects) or agnosia (difficulty recognizing familiar people).
Delusions	Common, fleeting, usually transient and poorly organized.	Often absent.
Hallucinations	Common and usually visual, tactile, and olfactory.	Often absent.
Speech	Often uncharacteristic, loud, rapid, or slow (hypoactive).	Difficulty in finding words and articulating thoughts; aphasia.
Affect	Mood liability.	Mood liability.
Sleep-wake cycle	Disturbed; may be reversed.	Can be fragmented.
Psychomotor activity	Increased, reduced, or unpredictable; variable depending on hyperdelirium or hypodelirium.	Can be normal; may exhibit apraxia.

Source: Adapted from Milisen K, Braes T, Fick D, et al. Cognitive assessment and differentiating the 3 Ds (dementia, depression, delirium). *Nurs Clin North Am.* 2006;41:1–22.

examination and the writing and drawing questions included in it may be cumbersome and difficult to perform in a palliative care population. A subset of four items from the MMSE may be adequate to screen for delirium and cognitive impairment: current year, date, backward spelling, and copy a design.[12]

Table 1.4 provides an overview of the instruments used to assess delirium. These instruments are reviewed because they distinguish delirium from dementia and assess at least several of the multiple features of delirium. Although all of these instruments require further study to determine application across varied settings and among different patient populations, the

Table 1.3 Cancer-Specific Risk Factors for Delirium

Type of Physiologic Risk Factor	Cancer-Specific Considerations
Nutritional deficiencies B vitamins Vitamin C Hypoproteinemia	• Symptom distress: nausea, emesis, mucositis, diarrhea, pain, and anorexia or cachexia syndrome • Surgical alteration of the head and neck region or gastrointestinal tract • Nonoral feeding routes: gastrostomy feeding tube and use of total parenteral nutrition
Cardiovascular abnormalities Decreased cardiac output states: myocardial infarction, dysrhythmias, congestive heart failure, and cardiogenic shock Alterations in peripheral vascular resistance: increased and decreased states Vascular occlusion: emboli and disseminated intravascular coagulopathy	• Septic shock syndrome • Hypercoagulopathy and hyperviscosity • Anthracycline-related cardiomyopathy • Central line occlusion • Thrombi associated with immobility and paraneoplastic syndromes • Disseminated intravascular coagulopathy
Cerebral disease Vascular insufficiency: transient ischemic attacks, cerebral vascular accidents, and thrombosis Central nervous system infection: acute or chronic meningitis, brain abscess, and neurosyphilis Trauma: subdural hematoma, contusion, concussion, and intracranial hemorrhage	• Intracerebral bleed caused by thrombocytopenia • Meningeal carcinomatosis • Central nervous system edema secondary to brain malignancy or whole brain radiation therapy • Fall risk • Malignancy: primary or metastatic involving brain and cranial irradiation
Endocrine disturbance Hypothyroidism Diabetes mellitus Hypercalcemia Hyponatremia Hypopituitarism	• Mantle field radiation therapy • Steroid induced • Related to bone metastases • Syndrome of inappropriate antidiuretic hormone, rigorous hydration, and dehydration • Brain tumor in or adjacent to pituitary gland
Temperature regulation fluctuation Hypothermia Hyperthermia	• Absence of customary warm clothes • Fever
Pulmonary abnormalities Inadequate gas-exchange states: pulmonary disease and alveolar hypoventilation Infection: pneumonia	• Hypoxemia • Anemia • Lung metastases • Bleomycin-induced pulmonary fibrosis • Radiotherapy to chest • Chest tubes • Neutropenia and immobility

(continued)

Table 1.3 (Continued)

Type of Physiologic Risk Factor	Cancer-Specific Considerations
Systemic infective process (acute or chronic) Viral Fungal Bacterial: endocarditis, pyelonephritis, and cystitis	• Prominence of neutropenia • Steroids • Hypogammaglobulinemia
Metabolic disturbance Electrolyte abnormalities: hypercalcemia, hyponatremia and hypernatremia, hypokalemia and hyperkalemia, hypocalcemia and hypercalcemia, and hyperphosphatemia Acidosis and alkalosis Hypoglycemia and hyperglycemia Acute and chronic renal failure Volume depletion: hemorrhage, inadequate fluid intake, diuretics, and diarrhea Hepatic failure	• Syndrome of inappropriate antidiuretic hormone • Bone metastases • Diabetes secondary to steroids • Renal malignancy • Dehydration and diarrhea secondary to pelvic radiotherapy or chemotherapy • Liver primary or metastases with ascites or encephalopathy • Tumor lysis syndrome
Drug intoxication (therapeutic or substance abuse) Misuse of prescribed medications Side effects of therapeutic medications Drug—drug interactions Drug—herb interactions Improper use of over-the-counter medications Alcohol intoxication or withdrawal	• Polypharmacy with drugs having anticholinergic or central nervous system effects • Inadequate knowledge about geriatric-specific pharmacokinetic considerations in dosing • Self-medication with over-the-counter or herbal remedies in the absence of healthcare professional awareness • Alcohol withdrawal perioperatively in patients with head and neck cancer

Source: Boyle D. Delirium in older adults with cancer: Implications for practice and research. *Oncol Nurs Forum*. 2006;33:61-78.

following have shown good reliability and validity in identifying delirium in selected populations:

- The Memorial Delirium Assessment Scale (MDAS) is a 10-item tool based on the DSM-IV criteria (which are consistent with the DSM-5 criteria) designed to quantify the severity of delirium.[13] It takes about 10 minutes to administer. The MDAS requires minimal training for use and is appropriate for both clinical practice and research.
- The Delirium Rating Scale (DRS) is a 10-item scale and the Delirium Rating Scale—Revised-98 (DRS-R98) is a 16-item scale. Both are intended to be used by clinicians with psychiatric training. The scales look at symptoms over a 24-hour period and maybe used to assess severity of delirium.[13]
- The Confusion Assessment Method (CAM) is based on the DSM-IV criteria for delirium and is designed for use by a trained interviewer to assess

Table 1.4 Overview of Delirium Assessment Tools

	MDAS	DRS	CAM	NCS	BCS	DOS	Nu-DESC
DSM-IV criterion							
Acute onset		X	X			X	X
Fluctuating nature		X	X			X	X
Physical disorder		X	X				
Consciousness	X		X		X	X	X
Attention/ concentration	X		X	X	X	X	
Thinking	X	X	X	X	X	X	X
Disorientation	X		X	X		X	X
Memory	X	X	X	X	X	X	
Perception	X	X	X			X	X
Purpose							
Screening/diagnosis		X	X	X	X	X	X
Symptom severity	X	X					
Number of items	10	10	9	9	2	13	5
Time to complete (minutes)	10	Not specified	<5	10	<2	5	1

BCS, Bedside Confusion Scale; CAM, Confusion Assessment Method; DOS, Delirium Observation Scale; DRS, Delirium Rating Scale; MDAS, Memorial Delirium Assessment Scale; NCS, NEECHAM Confusion Scale; Nu-DESC, Nursing Delirium Screening Scale.

cognitive functioning in elderly patients on a daily scheduled basis. The CAM and the CAM-ICU (revised for use in the intensive care unit setting) have been evaluated in a number of studies and show good reliability and validity.[12] A related tool, the Family Confusion Assessment Method (FAM-CAM), is designed to get family caregiver assessments and has been shown to correlate with a formal CAM evaluation.

- Nurses designed the NEECHAM Confusion Scale (NCS) for rapid and unobtrusive assessment and monitoring of acute confusion in hospitalized elderly patients.[14] It contains nine scaled items divided into three subscales and takes about 10 minutes to complete. The NCS has been studied in many populations, including nonintubated patients in intensive care units.[14]
- The Bedside Confusion Scale (BCS) consists of observation of the level of consciousness and timed recitation of the months of the year in reverse order starting with December and is designed for use in the palliative care setting. It requires minimal training and only about 2 minutes to complete. The BCS was found to correlate with the CAM, but it is subject to bias or inappropriate interpretation and has a limited capacity to assess the multiple cognitive domains influenced by delirium.
- The Delirium Observation Screening Scale (DOSS) is based on the DSM-IV criteria and is designed to assist nurses in the early recognition of delirium during routine care. The original version of the scale has 25 items. After

studies on geriatric and hip fracture patients, the scale was reduced to 13 items that can be rated as present or absent in less than 5 minutes.

- The Nursing Delirium Screening Scale (Nu-DESC) is an observational five-item instrument designed to be completed in about 1 minute at the beside.[15] It has been shown to have validity and sensitivity comparable to the MDAS in oncology populations and is a sensitive test in the recovery room to detect delirium.

Given the fluctuating nature of delirium, every-shift assessments in hospital and nursing home settings, using a simple screening tool such as the CAM, BCS, DOSS, or Nu-DESC, are appropriate, especially for high-risk populations. There are no published recommendations on the frequency with which delirium assessment tools should be used in outpatient and home care settings. Too-frequent evaluation for delirium in persons at low risk is burdensome to both the patient and the clinician. It makes sense to complete a baseline evaluation on all patients, and then base the frequency of follow-up assessments on the number of risk factors present for delirium. Simply asking the family, "Do you think [the patient] has been more confused lately?" may serve as a clinical screening tool to determine which patients require a more thorough evaluation.

Nursing Care of Persons at Risk for Experiencing Delirium

Optimal care of the person at risk for, or experiencing, delirium requires application of evidence-based practice guidelines by an interdisciplinary team that includes both palliative care bedside nurses and advanced practice nurses (APNs). The plan of care must align with the patient and family goals of care. Creation of the plan of care is initiated by the palliative care nurse with the guidance of the palliative care team. The plan should be both proactive, to prevent delirium when possible, and focused on alleviation of suffering for both patient and family. The following management guidelines address interventions appropriate for all types of delirium that commonly occur in patients with serious medical conditions: hyperactive, hypoactive, and mixed-type, as well as irreversible delirium that may occur at the end of life. Death-bed phenomena are discussed as a separate syndrome.

Evidenced-based guidelines focus on primary prevention by implementing risk prevention measures, using reliable and valid delirium screening and assessment tools, and addressing contributing factors for delirium for all patients with serious or advanced medical conditions. Figure 1.1 illustrates a suggested care pathway.

Strategies to Prevent and Mitigate Delirium

The correlation between the number of risk factors and the incidence of delirium suggests that a proactive plan of care may reduce the severity of a delirious episode or possibly prevent an acute delirious episode. Five risk

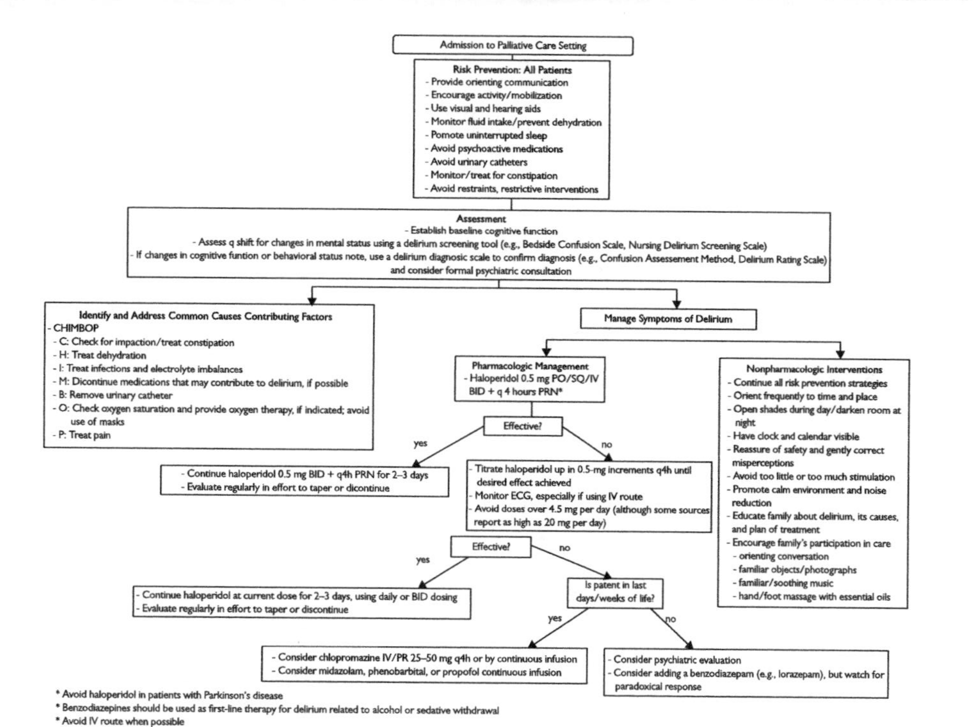

Figure 1.1 Delirium algorithm. ECG, electrocardiogram.

factors are predictive of delirium in the elderly hospitalized patient: physical restraints, malnutrition, three medications recently added, indwelling urinary catheter, and any recent medical event such as admission to an emergency room.

The American College of Critical Care Medicine published revised guidelines for the management of pain, agitation, and delirium in the intensive care unit setting in 2013.[16] These guidelines, often referred to as the "PAD bundle," emphasize (1) frequent reorientation and ensuring access to eyeglasses and hearing aids, if needed; (2) maintaining patients' sleep-wake cycles by minimizing environmental and procedural disturbances at night; and (3) advancing patients' mobility during the day as tolerated, with the goal of getting patients out of bed each day, even when they are intubated and mechanically ventilated.[16]

The palliative nursing plan of care includes ensuring frequent orientation, normalizing sleep routines, mobilizing the patient, engaging the patient in mentally stimulating activities, maintaining consistent and familiar caregivers, ensuring use of eyeglasses and hearing aids, monitoring fluid and food intake, and monitoring bowel function. Evaluation of and interventions to improve sleep quality cannot be overemphasized because this is both a contributing factor for delirium and one of the earliest signs of a developing delirium.

Despite an excellent plan of care that eliminates or minimizes risk factors, delirium may not be preventable in the final stages of life. The nurse must have a thorough knowledge of the patient's primary diagnosis, comorbidities, symptoms, prior activity, cognitive status, nutritional status, and prognosis. The physical examination rules out infectious, metabolic, endocrine, cardiovascular, and cerebrovascular disease that could contribute to delirium. This information, along with identifying medications that could contribute to delirium, alerts the palliative care team to patients who are at high risk for delirious episodes. Sedative hypnotics, opioids, medications with anticholinergic effects, benzodiazepines, and the use of multiple medications are all potential precipitating factors for delirium.[4] With the help of an interdisciplinary review, the medication profile can be streamlined.

Management of Acute Delirium

When delirium is present, a detailed workup is essential to identify the underlying cause, when possible. Laboratory examinations include compete blood count, blood urea nitrogen, and creatinine levels, liver function, and thyroid function. If an infectious process is suspected, urine culture, chest x-ray, and, possibly, arterial blood gases are evaluated. Serum vitamin B_{12} and folate levels may reveal nutritional imbalances. Brain imaging and scans could be of value when other more common causes have been ruled out because several advanced illness pathologies may extended to the brain (e.g., cancer and AIDS), causing an acute delirium. All laboratory and imaging tests are initiated only after consideration of what impact the information will have on the plan of care and if the tests are consistent with patient and family goals.[4] For example, if brain metastasis is suspected and the patient would not be a candidate for, or does not want, additional treatment, a brain scan would not be appropriate.

The acronym CHIMBOP can assist the nurse to rule out seven common causes of delirium.[17] While this tool does not address all of the potentially reversible causes of delirium, it provides a framework for nurses to begin searching for the etiologies of the delirium.

- C = Constipation—check for impaction; obtain order for and administer bowel stimulants and stool softeners.
- H = Hypovolemia, hypoglycemia—encourage oral intake or provide parenteral fluids; treat hypoglycemia.
- I = Infection—evaluate for signs and symptoms of infection; contact the physician or APN to determine whether anti-infective medications are appropriate at this time.
- M = Medications—review the patient's medications for those known to contribute to delirium; discuss minimizing or discontinuing medications, as possible, with the physician, APN, and pharmacist.
- B = Bladder catheter, bladder outlet obstruction—avoid the use of or remove urinary catheters; check for bladder distention and insert catheter (straight or indwelling) only if required.
- O = Oxygen deficiency—check oxygen saturation or signs of hypoxia and administer oxygen as indicated.
- P = Pain—evaluate for and treat pain.

Although dehydration is a documented contributing factor for delirium, artificial hydration is not necessarily helpful. A thorough evaluation of the patient's overall condition is necessary to determine whether a trial of artificial hydration is indicated. In addition, careful monitoring is required to ensure that the patient does not experience any uncomfortable symptoms associated with overhydration if artificial hydration is initiated.

Additional measures include providing a safe, quiet, and comforting environment for the patient. If the patient is in an area of high activity, either in the home or hospital, moving the patient to a quiet location may help. Eliminate extraneous noises such as televisions and intercoms that may stimulate the overtaxed brain. And, involve the family. The voice of a family member or significant other or the touch of the hand can communicate understanding and reassurance to the patient.

Physical restraints should be avoided whenever possible. Restraints should be used only when a patient poses a clear risk for harm to self or others. A better way to ensure patient safety is to arrange for one-on-one observation of the patient. Not only does one-on-one observation promote safety but also the presence of a trusted person may reduce the patient's anxiety and provide orientation cues. This person becomes part of the treatment plan for delirium.

An acute phase of delirium can last for hours or days. Following resolution of the acute phase of delirium, the nurse should continue assessments and delirium screenings because the patient remains at high risk for a reoccurrence of delirium. In the postdelirium state, it is important to debrief patients about what they remember. As mentioned previously, patients may recall distressing images or feel embarrassed about their behavior. Debriefing the experience can help patients and caregivers to normalize the event and reduce any stigma that patients may feel about being out of control and seemingly unaware of their behavior.

Management of Death-Bed Phenomena

As discussed earlier, death-bed phenomena are usually not distressing to patients. Therefore, a nonpharmacologic approach may be the most beneficial. Yet, these behaviors may create some concern on the part of the caregivers who wonder how to respond to the patient who is seeing and speaking to someone not visible to others.

The palliative care team can guides caregivers in listening carefully to the patient's words as they describe their visions. Often, a theme emerges in phrases, such as, "please open the door," "I will be home soon," or "I will catch the next train." The nurse can normalize the event by explaining that these experiences are common and that they indicate the patient is preparing for death. Additionally, the nurse can teach the family responses that may be helpful, such as, "The door is open, so you can go on when you are ready"; "We will miss you, but you can go when it's time"; "They are waiting and will be happy to see you"; or, "It is okay to catch the next train." The nurse and spiritual caregivers reframe the experience as a sacred passage for the patient, when family and loved ones are offered a time to say good-bye.

Pharmacologic Interventions for the Management of Delirium

Nonpharmacologic approaches and interventions to treat or lessen risk factors causing delirium are the first-line treatments for this syndrome.[4] No medications have been approved by the U.S. Food and Drug Administration (FDA) for the treatment of delirium, but when pharmacologic agents are required, antipsychotic agents are the medications of choice.[4] However, the use of antipsychotics for the treatment of delirium is not without controversy. Some clinicians feel that pharmacologic management should be used only for patients who have severe agitation that interferes with medical treatments or for patients who pose a danger to themselves. This approach means that those with hypoactive delirium rarely receive antipsychotics. Others suggest that pharmacologic interventions should be considered in all patients with delirium, especially those who have agitation, paranoia, hallucination, or altered sensorium, because of the distressing nature of these symptoms. Additional support for using antipsychotics for more than the severely agitated is that these medications have been shown to improve both arousal disturbance and impaired cognitive functioning in patients with hypoactive delirium.[4] In addition, current evidence does not indicate a difference in response rates between clinical subtypes of delirium. Clinicians who choose to take a "wait-and-see" approach before using antipsychotics for the delirious patient who is not agitated or having distressing hallucinations should be prepared to act quickly because the hypoactive, somnolent patient can become agitated very quickly. What is clear from the literature is that there is a wide range of prescribing patterns in the use of antipsychotics to manage delirium. Table 1.5 provides an overview of the more common medications used to treat delirium.

Haloperidol has fewer anticholinergic side effects, is less sedating, and has fewer active metabolites than other typical antipsychotics. There are few data to support the optimal dose or route of administration of haloperidol for delirium, and little is known about the optimal duration of treatment. Typical starting doses are 1 to 2 mg (oral, intramuscularly, intravenously, subcutaneously) for mild agitation, 5 mg for moderate agitation, and 7.5 to 10 mg for severe agitation. In elderly patients, lower doses (e.g., 0.25 to 0.5 mg) may be sufficient. Doses are repeated every 30 minutes until the patient is calm but arouses to normal voice.[4] When symptoms are controlled, the total dose given in the last 24 hours is given once per day or divided for twice-daily administration. Doses above 20 mg per day are not recommended, but doses as high as 250 mg in 24 hours have been used.[4] Generally, after 2 to 3 days with no evidence of delirium, the medication can be weaned while evaluating for return of symptoms. Ideally, during this time other interventions to address the underlying cause of delirium are also used. Long-term use of antipsychotics for persistent delirium has not been studied and increases both the risk for adverse events and costs.

Haloperidol can be given by the oral, sublingual, rectal, subcutaneous, intramuscular, or intravenous routes. Parenteral doses are approximately twice as potent as oral doses. The oral route is associated with more frequent extrapyramidal side effects than the intravenous route, but the intravenous route is not without problems.[18] Haloperidol can prolong the QTc interval and has been associated with torsades de points (TdP), especially when given intravenously or in higher doses than recommended. In 2007, the FDA issued an alert warning that cases of sudden death, TdP, and QTc prolongation have been reported even in the absence of predisposing factors; this warning included a reminder that haloperidol is not approved for intravenous administration and recommended electrocardiographic monitoring if it is given intravenously. Monitoring of QTc intervals is recommended before long-term, high-dose antipsychotic therapy, and there is some support for not initiating treatment with haloperidol administration if the QTc interval is greater than 450 msec. Weckmann and Morrison, in their review of the evidence, concluded that the choice to obtain an electrocardiogram should be based on the patient's overall condition, prognosis, expected mortality, distress level, and goals of care and that the benefits of treating delirium outweigh the risks.[18]

Chlorpromazine is another typical antipsychotic that may be used to treat delirium. Doses of 25 to 50 mg by the oral, sublingual, or parenteral route may be used.[4] Chlorpromazine is associated with more anticholinergic side effects, orthostatic hypotension, and sedation than haloperidol. Therefore, it is usually used only when the additional sedation will be of benefit and haloperidol has not been completely effective.

Table 1.5 Pharmacologic Treatment of Delirium

Class and Drug	Starting Dose and Titration	Usual Daily Dose	Comments
Typical Antipsychotic			
• Haloperidol	0.5 to 2 mg PO/SL/SQ/IM/IV every 30 min until settled, then up to 20 mg daily given in one or two divided doses, based on dose needed to settle	1 to 5 mg over 24 hr	• Most commonly used and studied medication for delirium • EPS, especially if dose is > 4.5 mg PO per day • Monitor QTc interval • Due to long half-life may be able to dose once daily after effective dose established
• Chlorpromazine	25 to 50 mg PO/SL/PR/IM/SQ/IV every 1 hr until settled, then 25 to 100 mg 6 to 8 hr ATC or PRN, based on dose needed to settle	PO: 50 mg tid SQ: 5 to 50 mg/hr	• Useful if a more sedating agent is desired • Higher risk for anticholinergic side effects than with haloperidol • Monitor blood pressure for orthostatic hypotension • If using IV route, give by slow push or infusion over 10 to 15 minutes
Atypical Antipsychotic			**Class characteristics:** • EPS equivalent to or slightly less than those of haloperidol • Prolonged QTc interval • More expensive than typical antipsychotics
• Olanzapine	2.5 to 5 mg PO daily, may increase to 10 mg daily	5 mg bid	• Available in orally disintegrating tablets

• Risperidone	0.25 to 0.5 mg PO twice daily and PRN; may increase by 0.5 mg every other day	1 mg bid	• Available in orally disintegrating tablets • Monitor blood pressure for orthostatic hypotension
• Quetiapine	12.5 to 25 mg PO twice daily; may give 12.5 mg in morning and 25 mg at night, increasing as necessary	50 mg bid	• Most sedating of this class • Preferred agent in patients with Parkinson's disease • Monitor blood pressure for orthostatic hypotension
Benzodiazepine			
• Lorazepam	0.5 to 1 mg PO/IV every 4 hr PRN		• Often worsens delirium • Sedating, but can see paradoxical excitation • Medication of choice in patients with delirium associated with sedative or alcohol withdrawal or those with neuroleptic malignant syndrome • Second-line agent for delirium in patients with Parkinson's disease

ATC, around the clock; EPS, extrapyramidal symptoms; IV, intravenous; PO, oral; PR, rectal; SL, sublingual; SQ, subcutaneous; PRN, as needed.

Sources: Irwin S, Pirreilo RD, Hirst JM, Buckholz GT, Ferris FD. Clarifying delirium management: practical, evidenced-based, expert recommendations for clinical practice. *J Palliat Med.* 2013;16:423–435; and Weckmann MT, Morrison RS. What pharmacological treatments are effective for delirium? In: Goldstein NE, Morrison RS, eds. *Evidence-Based Practice of Palliative Medicine*. Philadelphia: Elsevier; 2013:205–210.

Atypical antipsychotics have the advantage of fewer extrapyramidal side effects and less effect on QTc interval.[4] None of these medications is approved by the FDA for the treatment of delirium, and all of them are more expensive than haloperidol. With the exception of olanzapine, these drugs do not come in a parenteral form. Studies support that haloperidol, risperidone, olanzapine, and quetiapine are equally effective in treating delirium with few adverse events.[4] Starting doses are outlined in Table 1.5. First-generation antipsychotics (i.e., haloperidol and chlorpromazine) are considered first-line therapy, unless the patient has Parkinson's disease, in which case quetiapine is recommended.

Cholinesterase inhibitors have been studied for the treatment of delirium based on the understanding that disruption of the cholinergic system may be one of the underlying mechanisms of this syndrome. However, there is currently no evidence from controlled trials that the cholinesterase inhibitors are effective in the treatment of delirium.[19]

Benzodiazepines are not recommended as the first-line treatment of delirium, except for delirium associated with alcohol or sedative-hypnotic drug withdrawal.[4] This class of medications tends to cause oversedation and exacerbate confusion, potentially making delirium worse. If haloperidol does not control the agitation of delirium, the clinician may consider switching to chlorpromazine or adding a benzodiazepine, most frequently lorazepam.[4] The patient must be monitored carefully to ensure that the addition of the benzodiazepine does not make the delirium worse. Irwin and colleagues suggest that if paradoxical agitation occurs with lorazepam, rapid titration of lorazepam to higher doses will usually overcome this reaction and palliate symptoms.[4] Some clinicians will avoid benzodiazepines and treat this as a refractory delirium.

Family and Caregiver Education and Support

Family and caregiver education about delirium and its associated risk factors is essential because caregiver assistance is needed to maintain daily routines, decrease risk factors that precipitate delirium, and identify early signs and symptoms of delirium. Watching a loved one spiral into confusion and paranoia is overwhelming to caregivers. Caregivers require education and support to respond to their dying loved one's agitation or sudden withdrawal into silence. Psychosocial and spiritual care are essential components of the continuum of support for the caregivers' journey with illness and death. A simple inquiry from the nurse to the caregiver, "tell me what this is like for you," provides the opportunity for caregivers to express their needs for support as well as the anguish over seeing a loved one decline physically and mentally.

The goals of caregiver education depend on where the patient resides (home, residential or acute care) and the stage of the patient's chronic or terminal illness (beginning, middle, end). Consideration is given to caregivers' ethnicity, level of education, and the resources available in the care setting. Education can be directed toward understanding delirium and its possible causes, ways to communicate with the patient (including while ventilated), orientation methods, and how to comfort the patient with touch, familiar sounds, and other sensory aids. Nurses can facilitate referrals to chaplains and social workers, who may be available to offer additional support. Written information is helpful for reinforcing education. As an example, a "Quick Reference Sheet" about delirium is available in English and Spanish from the Hospice and Palliative Nurses Association.[20]

References

1. Hosie A, Davidson PM, Agar M, Sanderson CR, Phillips J. Delirium prevalence, incidence, and implications for screening in specialist palliative care inpatient settings: a systematic review. *Palliat Med*. 2012;27:486–498.
2. Wand AP, Thoo W, Ting V, Baker J, Sciuriaga H, Hunt GE. Identification and rates of delirium in elderly medical inpatients from diverse language groups. *Geriatr Nurs*. 2013;34:355–360.
3. Grover S, Shah R. Distress due to delirium experience. *Gen Hosp Psychiatry*. 2011;33:637–639.
4. Irwin S, Pirreilo RD, Hirst JM, Buckholz GT, Ferris FD. Clarifying delirium management: practical, evidenced-based, expert recommendations for clinical practice. *J Palliat Med*. 2013;16:423–435.
5. American Psychiatric Association. *Diagnostic and Statistical Manual of Mental Disorders (DSM-5)*. Arlington, VA: American Psychiatric Association; 2013.
6. Chirco N, Dunn KS, Robinson SG. The trajectory of terminal delirium at the end of life. *J Hosp Palliat Nurs*. 2011;13:411–418.
7. Mazzarino-Willett A. Deathbed phenomena: its role in peaceful death and terminal restlessness. *Am J Hosp Palliat Care*. 2010;27:127–133.
8. Callanan C, Kelley P. *Final Gifts*. New York: Poseidon Press; 1992:67–71.
9. Inouye S. Delirium in older persons. *N Engl J Med*. 2006;354:1157–1165.
10. Milisen K, Braes T, Fick D, et al. Cognitive assessment and differentiating the 3 Ds (dementia, depression, delirium). *Nurs Clin North Am*. 2006;41:1–22.
11. Boyle D. Delirium in older adults with cancer: Implications for practice and research. *Oncol Nurs Forum*. 2006;33:61–78.
12. Morandi A, McCurley J, Vasilevskis EE, Fick DM. Tools to detect delirium superimposed on dementia: a systematic review. *J Am Geriatr Soc*. 2012;60:2005–2013.
13. Wong CL, Holroyd-Leduc J, Simel DL, Straus SE. Does this patient have delirium? Value of bedside instruments. *JAMA*. 2010;304:779–786.
14. Matarese M, Generoso S, Ivziku D, Pedone C, DeMarinis MG. Delirium in older patients: a diagnostic study of NEECHAM Confusion Scale in surgical intensive care unit. *J Clin Nurs*. 2013;22:2849–2857.
15. Gaudreau J, Gagnon P, Harel F, et al. Fast, systematic, and continuous delirium assessment in hospitalized patients: the nursing delirium screening scale. *J Pain Symptom Manage*. 2005;29:368–375.
16. Barr J, Pandharipande PP. The pain, agitation, and delirium care bundle: synergistic benefits of implementing the 2013 pain, agitation, and delirium guidelines in an integrated and interdisciplinary fashion. *Crit Care Med*. 2013;41:S99–S115.
17. Zama I, Maynard W, Davis M. Clocking delirium: the value of the clock drawing test with case illustrations. *Am J Hosp Palliat Care*. 2008;25:385–388.

18. Weckmann MT, Morrison RS. What pharmacological treatments are effective for delirium? In: Goldstein NE, Morrison RS, eds. *Evidence-Based Practice of Palliative Medicine*. Philadelphia: Elsevier; 2013:205–210.

19. Overshott R, Karim S, Burns A. Cholinesterase inhibitors for delirium. *Cochrane Database Syst Rev.* 2008(1);CD005317.

20. Hospice and Palliative Nurses Association. Quick reference sheet: delirium in hospice and palliative patients. Revised 7/2013. Available at http://www.hpna.org/DisplayPage.aspx?Title=Quick%20Information%20Sheet (accessed December 3, 2013).

Chapter 2

Dyspnea, Death Rattle, and Cough

Deborah Dudgeon

Dyspnea

Dyspnea is a common symptom in people with advanced disease and can severely impair their quality of life. Management of dyspnea requires understanding and assessment of the multidimensional components of the symptom, knowledge of the pathophysiologic mechanisms and clinical syndromes that are common in people with advanced disease, and knowledge of the indications and limitations of the available therapeutic approaches.

Definition

Dyspnea, like pain, is multidimensional in nature, with not only physical elements but also affective components, which are shaped by previous experience.[1] A neurophysiologic model provides a framework to understand the variety of mechanisms that can lead to dyspnea: receptor → afferent impulse → integration/processing in the central nervous system (CNS) → efferent impulse → dyspnea.[1] Stimulation of a number of different receptors (Figure 2.1), and the conscious perception this stimulation invokes, can alter ventilation and result in both the intensity and unpleasantness sensations of breathlessness.[1]

Prevalence and Impact

The prevalence of dyspnea varies according to the stage and type of underlying disease and the methodologic design of the studies.[2] A systematic review of symptom prevalence in advanced cancer, AIDS, heart disease, chronic obstructive pulmonary disease (COPD), and renal disease found that the prevalence of dyspnea was 10% to 70% in patients with cancer, 11% to 62% in patients with AIDS, 60% to 88% in those with heart disease, 90% to 95% in those with COPD, and 11% to 62% in patients renal disease.[2]

In a consecutive cohort of 5862 patients seen by a specialist palliative care service during a 4-year period, dyspnea was evaluated at every clinical encounter until death. Only 11.4% of people had "no breathlessness" recorded between referral and death. Patients with noncancer causes of breathlessness had significantly higher levels for the last 3 months of life with no significant changes. Cancer patients had significantly lower levels of breathlessness initially, but the intensity worsened between 3 and 10 days

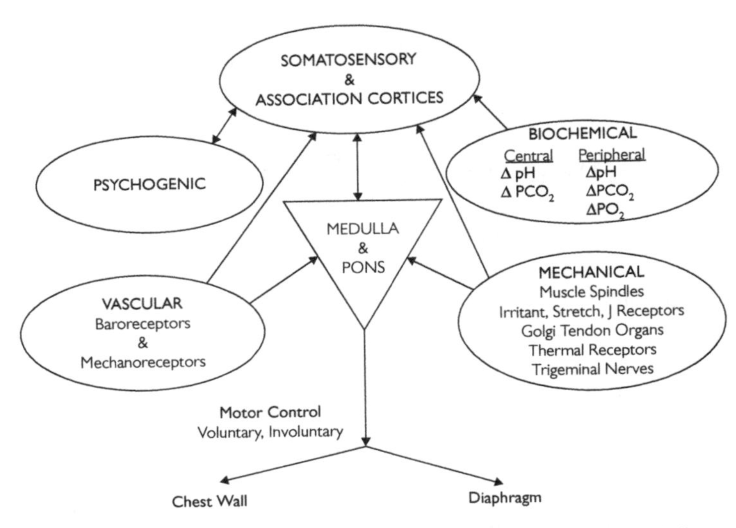

Figure 2.1 Schematic diagram of the neuroanatomic elements involved in the control of ventilation.

before death. Despite symptomatic treatment at death, 65% of people were breathless, and it was severe in 26% of the individuals.[3]

Patients with advanced disease typically experience chronic shortness of breath with intermittent acute episodes. Acute attacks of breathlessness are usually accompanied by feelings of anxiety, fear, panic, and, if severe enough, a sensation of impending death.[1] Many dying persons are terrified of waking in the middle of the night with intense air hunger. They need providers who will anticipate their fears and provide symptomatic relief of their breathlessness and anxiety as they approach death.

Pathophysiology

Management of dyspnea requires an understanding of its multidimensional nature and the pathophysiologic mechanisms that cause this distressing symptom. Exertional dyspnea in cardiopulmonary disease (Box 2.1) is caused by increased ventilatory demand, impaired mechanical responses, or a combination of the two. The effects of abnormalities of these mechanisms can also be additive.

Multidimensional Assessment of Dyspnea

Dyspnea, like pain, is a subjective experience that may not be evident to an observer. *Tachypnea*, a rapid respiratory rate, is not dyspnea. Medical personnel must learn to ask for and accept the patient's assessments, often without measurable physical correlates. If patients say they are having discomfort with breathing, we must believe that they are dyspneic.

To determine whether dyspnea is present, it is important to ask more than the question, "Are you short of breath?" Patients often respond in the negative to this simple question because they have limited their activities so that

Box 2.1 Pathophysiologic Mechanisms of Dyspnea

Increased Ventilatory Demand

Increased physiologic dead space
- Thromboemboli
- Tumor emboli
- Vascular obstruction
- Radiation therapy
- Chemotherapy
- Emphysema

Severe deconditioning
Hypoxemia
Change in V_{CO_2} or arterial P_{CO_2} set point
Psychological: anxiety, depression
Increased neural reflex activity

Impaired Mechanical Response or Ventilatory Pump

Restrictive ventilatory deficit
Respiratory muscle weakness
- Cachexia
- Electrolyte imbalances
- Peripheral muscle weakness
- Neuromuscular abnormalities
- Neurohumoral
- Steroids

Pleural or parenchymal disease
Reduced chest wall compliance
Obstructive ventilatory deficit
Asthma
Chronic obstructive pulmonary disease
Tumor obstruction
Mixed obstructive and restrictive disorder (any combination of the above)

they won't become short of breath. It is therefore helpful to ask about shortness of breath in relationship to activities:

"Do you get short of breath walking at the same speed as someone of your age?"
"Do you have to stop to catch your breath when walking upstairs?"
"Do you get short of breath when you are eating?"

Qualitative and Affective Aspects of Dyspnea

It is now recognized that dyspnea is not a single sensation. There are at least three different "qualities" of uncomfortable breathing: "air hunger," "work," and "tightness."[4] Each of these sensations is thought to arise from a different afferent source. Air hunger arises when pulmonary ventilation is insufficient and there is a conscious perception of the urge to breath. The sense of excessive work of breathing occurs when there is an increased rate or depth, impedance to inspiration, or respiratory muscle weakness or when there is a disadvantageous length of the respiratory muscles. Tightness is specific to bronchoconstriction.

Clinical Assessment

Clinical assessments are usually directed at determining the underlying pathophysiology, deciding appropriate treatment, and evaluating the response to therapy. The clinical assessment of dyspnea should include a complete history of the symptom, including its temporal onset (acute or chronic); whether it is affected by positioning; its qualities, associated symptoms, precipitation, and relieving events or activities; and its response to medications. A past history of smoking, underlying lung or cardiac disease, concurrent medical conditions, allergy history, and details of previous medications or treatments should be elicited. Assessment of the impact of breathlessness on the person's quality of life, physical activities, self-care, social life, and psychological state should also be undertaken.

Careful physical examination focused on possible underlying causes of dyspnea should be performed. Particular attention should be directed at signs associated with certain clinical syndromes that are common causes of dyspnea. Examples are dullness to percussion, decreased tactile fremitus, and absent breath sounds associated with a pleural effusion in a person with lung cancer; an elevated jugular venous pressure (JVP), audible third heart sound (S_3), and bilateral crackles audible on chest examination associated with congestive heart failure (CHF); and elevated JVP, distant heart sounds, and pulsus paradoxus in people with pericardial effusions.

Diagnostic tests helpful in determining the cause of dyspnea include chest radiography; electrocardiography; pulmonary function tests; arterial blood gases; complete blood counts; serum potassium, magnesium, and phosphate levels; cardiopulmonary exercise testing; and tests specific for suspected underlying pathologies, such as an echocardiogram for suspected pericardial effusion. The choice of appropriate diagnostic tests should be guided by the stage of disease, the prognosis, the risk-to-benefit ratios of any proposed tests or interventions, and the desires of the patient and family.

The Visual Analog Scale (VAS) is one of the most popular techniques for measuring the perceived intensity of dyspnea. This scale is usually a 100-mm vertical or horizontal line, anchored at each end by words such as "Not at all breathless" and "Very breathless." Subjects are asked to mark the line at the point that best describes the intensity of their breathlessness. The scales can be used as an initial assessment, to monitor progress, and to evaluate effectiveness of treatment in an individual patient. Numeric rating scales are highly correlated with VAS ratings of breathlessness and more repeatable measures that require a smaller sample size to detect a change in breathlessness.[5]

Dyspnea and Psychological Factors

The person's perception of the intensity of his or her breathlessness is also affected by psychological factors. Anxious, obsessive, depressed, and dependent persons appear to experience dyspnea that is disproportionately severe relative to the extent of their pulmonary disease.[1]

Management

The optimal treatment of dyspnea is to treat reversible causes. If this is no longer possible, then both pharmacologic and nonpharmacologic methods are used (Box 2.2).

Pharmacologic Interventions

Opioids

Since the late 19th century, opioids have been used to relieve breathlessness of patients with asthma, pneumothorax, and emphysema.[6] Although most trials have demonstrated the benefit of opioids for the treatment of dyspnea, some have been negative or have produced undesirable side effects.

Recent systematic reviews of the management of dyspnea in cancer patients also support the use of oral or parenteral opioids.[7,8]

In previous years, there was tremendous interest in the use of nebulized opioids for the treatment of dyspnea. Opioid receptors are present on sensory nerve endings in the airways; therefore it is hypothesized that if the receptors were interrupted directly, lower doses, with less systemic side effects, would be required to control breathlessness. Studies reveal no evidence that nebulized opioids are more effective than nebulized saline in relieving breathlessness. Given the results of these trials, it is hard to justify the continued use of nebulized opioids alone.

Physicians have been reluctant to prescribe opioids for dyspnea because of fears of respiratory failure. In studies of cancer patients, morphine did not compromise respiratory function as measured by respiratory effort and

Box 2.2 Management of Dyspnea

Pharmacologic Interventions

Chronic

Opioids

Add phenothiazine (chlorpromazine, promethazine)

Acute

Opioids

Add anxiolytic

Nonpharmacologic Interventions

Sit upright supported by pillows or leaning on overbed table

Fan with or without oxygen

Relaxation techniques and other appropriate nonpharmacologic measures

Identify and treat underlying diagnosis (if appropriate)

oxygen saturation or respiratory rate and $PaCO_2$. In another study, authors found the patients' intensity of dyspnea and respiratory rates decreased significantly ($P = 0.003$) after the administration of an opioid, but there was no significant change in the transcutaneous arterial pressure of CO_2.[9] It is now thought that the development of clinically significant hypoventilation and respiratory depression from opioids depends on the rate of change of the dose, the history of previous exposure to opioids, and possibly the route of administration. Early use of opioids improves quality of life and allows the use of lower doses, while tolerance to the respiratory depressant effects develops.

Sedatives and Tranquilizers

A systematic review examined whether benzodiazepines relieved breathlessness in adults with advanced disease. Seven studies with 200 subjects with advanced cancer or COPD were included in the analysis. No significant effect of benzodiazepines for relief of breathlessness or in the percentage of breakthrough dyspnea was observed.[10]

Combinations

In a randomized, single-blind 2-day study, dyspneic cancer patients were given routine subcutaneous doses of morphine, every 4 hours, with breakthrough midazolam; routine doses of midazolam with breakthrough morphine; or routine doses of both midazolam and morphine.[11] Significant improvements in dyspnea occurred in all three arms of the study. At 24 and 48 hours, significantly more patients who received the combined treatment of morphine and midazolam reported relief of dyspnea and had less episodes of breakthrough dyspnea with apparently no greater levels of sedation.

Oxygen

In hypoxic patients with COPD, oxygen supplementation improves survival, pulmonary hemodynamics, exercise capacity, and neuropsychological performance. Guidelines for oxygen use in this setting are shown in Box 2.3. The usefulness of oxygen to relieve breathlessness in the person with refractory dyspnea is less clear. In a Cochrane review to determine whether oxygen therapy provided relief of dyspnea in chronic end-stage disease, Cranston and colleagues[12] identified eight crossover studies that met their inclusion criteria. There were 144 participants (97 with cancer, 35 with cardiac failure and kyphoscoliosis).[12] In the patients with cancer, the meta-analysis failed to demonstrate a significant improvement of dyspnea at rest when oxygen was compared with air inhalation; improvement in dyspnea with oxygen inhalation was independent of resting hypoxia; and the patients perceived an improvement in dyspnea with inhalation of oxygen at rest and during exercise. In the participants with cardiac failure, high concentration of oxygen provided relief of dyspnea at 6 minutes during exercise tests, but low-flow ambulatory oxygen during a submaximal exercise test did not provide relief. In a single study of oxygen inhalation during exercise in the participants with kyphoscoliosis, oxygen improved dyspnea. The authors of this systematic review stated that their outcomes were inconclusive.[12] In a subsequent randomized, double-blind, crossover trial of the effect of oxygen versus air on the relief of dyspnea in 51 cancer patients, Philip and colleagues[13] found the mean sensation of dyspnea improved with both air and oxygen, with no

Box 2.3 Guidelines for Oxygen Therapy

Continuous oxygen:

PaO_2 ≤55 mm Hg or oxygen saturation ≤88% at rest

PaO_2 of 56 to 59 mm Hg or oxygen saturation of 89% in the presence of the following:

Dependent edema suggesting congestive heart failure

Cor pulmonale

Polycythemia (hematocrit >56%)

Pulmonary hypertension

Noncontinuous oxygen is recommended during exercise:

PaO_2 ≤55 mm Hg or oxygen saturation ≤88% with a low level of exertion, or during sleep

PaO_2 of ≤55 mm Hg or oxygen saturation ≤88% associated with pulmonary hypertension, daytime somnolence, and cardiac arrhythmias

significant differences in either VAS or patient preference between treatments. The 17 hypoxic patients also did not report a mean greater improvement with, or preference for, oxygen over air, despite improved oxygen saturations in all but 4 patients. The authors concluded that either air or oxygen via nasal prongs improved breathlessness.[13]

In a double-blind, controlled trial, 239 nonhypoxic individuals with a life-limiting illness were randomized to receive oxygen or room air for relief of dyspnea. Participants received air or oxygen by concentrator for at least 15 hours per day for 7 days, and breathlessness was measured twice a day. Oxygen did not provide additional benefit for relief of breathlessness compared with room air.[14]

Nonpharmacologic Interventions

Nonpharmacologic interventions for breathlessness may include sitting near an open window or in front of a stationary or handheld fan or having cold directed against the cheek or through the nose.

Nursing Interventions

Many patients obtain relief of dyspnea by leaning forward while sitting and supporting their upper arms on a table. Pursed-lip breathing slows the respiratory rate and increases intra-airway pressures, thus decreasing small airway collapse during periods of increased dyspnea. Nursing interventions may include teaching breathing retraining, relaxation, coping and adaptation strategies, muscle relaxation techniques, and guided imagery.

Patient and Family Teaching

Patients and families should be taught about the signs and symptoms of an impending exacerbation and how to manage the situation. They should learn problem-solving techniques to prevent panic, ways of conserving energy, how to prioritize activities, use of fans, and ways to maximize the effectiveness of their medications, such as using a spacer with inhaled drugs or taking an additional dose of an inhaled β-adrenergic agonist before exercise. Patients should avoid activities in which their arms are unsupported because these activities often increase breathlessness.

Patients in distress should not be left alone. Social services, nursing, and family input need to be increased as the patients' ability to care for themselves decreases.

Summary

Dyspnea is a common symptom in people with advanced disease. The symptom is often unrecognized, and patients therefore receive little assistance in managing their breathlessness. Dyspnea can have profound effects on a person's quality of life because even the slightest exertion may precipitate breathlessness.

Terminal Secretions

Noisy, rattling breathing in patients who are dying is commonly known as death rattle. This noisy, moist breathing can be distressing for the family, other patients, visitors, and healthcare workers because it may appear that the person is drowning in his or her own secretions. Management of death rattle can present healthcare providers with a tremendous challenge as they attempt to ensure a peaceful death for the patient.

Definition

Death rattle is a term applied to describe the noise produced by the turbulent movements of secretions in the upper airways that occur with the inspiratory and expiratory phases of respiration in patients who are dying.[15]

Prevalence and Impact

Death rattle occurs in 23% to 92% of patients in their last hours before death.[15] Studies have shown that there is an increased incidence of respiratory congestion in patients with primary lung cancer, cerebral metastases, pneumonia, and dysphagia, with the symptom more likely to persist in cases with pulmonary pathology. The incidence of death rattle increases closer to death; the median time from onset of death rattle to death is 8 to 23 hours.[16] Most commonly, this symptom occurs when the person's general condition is very poor, and most patients have a decreased level of consciousness. If the person is alert, however, the respiratory secretions can cause him or her to feel agitated and fearful of suffocating. A qualitative study involving hospice staff and volunteers found that most participants had negative feelings about hearing the sound of death rattle and thought that relatives were distressed by it as well.[17] Studies of bereaved relatives, however, found that not all were distressed by the sound, and this was, in part, determined by whether the person appeared disturbed or if they saw fluid dribbling from the person's mouth.

Assessment

Assessment of death rattle includes a focused history and physical examination to determine potentially treatable underlying causes. If the onset is sudden and is associated with acute shortness of breath and chest pain, it might suggest a pulmonary embolism or myocardial infarction. Physical findings consistent with CHF and fluid overload might support a trial of diuretic therapy; the presence of pneumonia indicates a trial of antibiotic therapy. The effectiveness of interventions should be included in the assessment. The patient's and family's understanding and emotional response to the situation should also be assessed so that appropriate interventions can be undertaken.

Management

Pharmacologic Interventions

Primary treatment should be focused on the underlying disorder, if appropriate to the prognosis and the wishes of the patient and family. If this is not possible, then anticholinergics are the primary mode of treatment.

Hyoscine hydrobromide (scopolamine), atropine sulfate, hyoscine butylbromide (Buscopan), and glycopyrrolate (Robinul) are the anticholinergic agents that are used to treat death rattle.

Hyoscine hydrobromide (scopolamine) is the primary medication used for the treatment of death rattle. It inhibits the muscarinic receptors and causes anticholinergic actions such as decreased peristalsis, gastrointestinal secretions, sedation, urinary retention, and dilation of the bronchial smooth muscle. It is administered subcutaneously, intermittently or by continuous infusion, orally, intravenously, or transdermally.

Atropine sulfate is another anticholinergic drug that is preferred by some centers for the treatment of respiratory congestion.[13] Atropine results in less CNS depression, delirium, and restlessness, with more bronchodilatory effect, than hyoscine hydrobromide. There is, however, the risk for increased tachycardia with atropine sulfate when doses higher than 1 mg are given. In one trial 137 participants were randomized to atropine or placebo. Sublingual atropine as a single dose was no more effective than placebo.[18]

Glycopyrrolate (Robinul) is also an anticholinergic agent. It has the advantages of producing less sedation and agitation and a longer duration of action than hyoscine hydrobromide. Glycopyrrolate is available in an oral form and

Box 2.4 Management of Death Rattle

Pharmacologic Interventions

Chronic

Glycopyrrolate or hyoscine hydrobromide patch

If treatment fails: Subcutaneous hyoscine hydrobromide or atropine sulfate

Acute

Subcutaneous hyoscine hydrobromide or subcutaneous atropine sulfate

Nonpharmacologic Interventions

Change position

Reevaluate if receiving intravenous hydration

can be useful for patients at an earlier stage of disease, when sedation is not desired.

Hyoscine butylbromide (Buscopan) is another anticholinergic drug. It is available in injection, suppository, and tablet forms.

Nonpharmacologic Interventions

There are times when the simple repositioning may help the patient to clear the secretions (Box 2.4). Suctioning usually is not recommended because it can be uncomfortable for the patient and causes significant agitation and distress. Pharmacologic measures are usually effective and prevent the need for suctioning. If the patient has copious secretions that can easily be reached in the oropharynx, then suctioning may be appropriate.

Patient and Family Teaching

The patient and the family can be distressed by this symptom. It is important to explain the process in order to help them understand why there is a buildup of secretions and that there is something that can be done to help. When explaining to families the changes that can occur before death, this is one of the symptoms that should be mentioned. If the person is being treated at home, the family should be instructed as to the measures available to relieve death rattle and to notify their hospice or palliative care team if it occurs so that appropriate medications can be ordered.

Summary

Although death rattle is a relatively common problem in people who are close to death, few studies have evaluated the effectiveness of treatment. Anticholinergics are the drugs of choice at this time. Death rattle can be distressing for family members at the bedside, and they need to receive good teaching and reassurance.

Cough

Cough is a natural defense of the body to prevent entry of foreign material into the respiratory tract. In people with advanced disease, it can be debilitating, leading to sleepless nights, fatigue, pain, and, at times, pathologic fractures.

Definition

Cough is an explosive expiration that can be a conscious act or a reflex response to an irritation of the tracheobronchial tree. Cough lasting 8 weeks is considered chronic. A *dry cough* occurs when no sputum is produced; a *productive cough* is one in which sputum is raised. *Hemoptysis* occurs when the sputum contains blood. *Massive hemoptysis* is expectoration of at least 100 to 600 mL of blood in 24 hours.

Prevalence and Impact

Chronic cough is a common problem in people with advanced diseases such as bronchitis, CHF, uncontrolled asthma, HIV infection, and various cancers. Cough can be precipitated by cold, smoke, a variety of smells, lying down, physical exertion, and some types of food. Cough may be distressing and can cause pain, fractured ribs, heaving, and retching and may reduce quality of life.

Assessment

In assessing someone with cough, it is important to undertake a thorough history and physical examination. Because cough may arise from anywhere in the distribution of the vagus nerve, the full assessment of a patient with a chronic cough requires a multidisciplinary approach with cooperation between respiratory medicine, gastroenterology, and ear, nose, and throat departments. The assessment helps to determine the underlying cause and appropriate treatment of the cough. Depending on the diagnosis, the prognosis, and the patient's and family's wishes, it may be appropriate to perform diagnostic tests, including chest or sinus radiography, spirometry before and after bronchodilator and histamine challenge, and, in special circumstances in people with earlier-stage disease, upper gastrointestinal endoscopy and 24-hour esophageal pH monitoring. In patients with significant hemoptysis, bronchoscopy is usually needed to identify the source of bleeding.

The history and physical examination should include assessment for a link between cough and the associated factors listed in the previous section, timing of the start of the cough, whether the cough is productive, whether the cough is nocturnal or daytime, the nature of the sputum, the frequency and amount of blood, precipitating and relieving factors, associated symptoms, and the effect on quality of life.[19]

Management

It is important to base management decisions on the cause and the appropriateness of treating the underlying diagnosis compared with simply suppressing the symptom. This decision is based on the diagnosis, prognosis, side effects, and possible benefits of the intervention and the wishes of the patient and family. Management strategies also depend on whether the cough is productive (Box 2.5) because cough suppressants, by causing mucus retention, could be harmful in conditions with excess mucus production.

Pharmacologic Interventions

There are three broad mechanisms of sensitization to cough relevant to treatments: peripheral sensitization, central sensitization, and impaired inhibition.

Centrally Acting Antitussives

Central Sensitization Central sensitization occurs when the central integrating neurons develop lower thresholds for activation in response to peripheral sensory stimulation. Upregulation of the *N*-methyl-D-aspartate (NMDA)

Box 2.5 Treatment of Nonproductive Cough

Nonopioid antitussive (dextromethorphan, benzonatate)
Opioids
Inhaled anesthetic (lidocaine, bupivacaine)

receptor is a postsynaptic mechanism that is critical to the initiation and maintenance of central sensitization.[20] Dextromethorphan, a dextro isomer of levorphanol, is an NMDA receptor antagonist that is almost equiantitussive to codeine. Dextromethorphan blocks the NMDA receptor to increase the cough threshold.

Opioids suppress cough, but the dose needed is higher than that contained in the proprietary cough mixtures. The exact mode of action is unclear, but it is thought that opioids inhibit the μ receptor peripherally in the lung; act centrally by suppressing the cough center in the medulla or the brainstem respiratory centers; or stimulate the μ receptor, thus decreasing mucus production or increasing mucus ciliary clearance. Codeine is the most widely used opioid for cough; some authors claim that it has no advantages over other opioids and provides no additional benefit to patients already receiving high doses of opioids for analgesia, whereas others state that the various opioids have different antitussive potencies.

Peripherally Acting Antitussives *Demulcents* are a group of compounds that form aqueous solutions and help to alleviate irritation of abraded surfaces. They are often found in over-the-counter cough syrups. Their mode of action for controlling cough is unclear, but it is thought that their sugar content encourages saliva production and swallowing, which leads to a decrease in the cough reflex; that they stimulate the sensory nerve endings in the epipharynx and decrease the cough reflex by a "gating" process; or that they may act as a protective barrier by coating the sensory receptors.

Benzonatate is an antitussive that inhibits cough mainly by anesthetizing the vagal stretch receptors in the bronchi, alveoli, and pleura. Other drugs that act directly on cough receptors include levodropropizine, oxalamine, and prenoxdiazine.[20] Inhaled anticholinergic *bronchodilators*, either alone or in combination with β_2-adrenergic agonists, effectively decrease cough in people with asthma and in normal subjects. It is thought that they decrease input from the stretch receptors, thereby decreasing the cough reflex, and change the mucociliary clearance.

The local anesthetic lidocaine is a nonselective voltage-gated sodium channel blocker that acts as a potent suppressor of irritant-induced cough and has been used as a topical anesthetic for the airway during bronchoscopy. *Inhaled local anesthetics*, such as lidocaine and bupivacaine, delivered by nebulizer, suppress some cases of chronic cough for as long as 9 weeks. Higher doses can cause bronchoconstriction, so it is wise to observe the first treatment. Patients must also be warned not to eat or drink anything for 1 hour after the treatment or until their cough reflex returns.

The leukotriene receptor antagonists montelukast and zafirlukast may reduce cough in cough-variant asthma. Menthol is thought to work through activation of a ligand-gated ion channel on sensory afferent fibers.

Productive Coughs

Interventions for productive coughs include chest physiotherapy, oxygen, humidity, and suctioning. In cases of increased sputum production, expectorants, mucolytics, and agents to decrease mucus production can be employed.

Opioids, antihistamines, and anticholinergics decrease mucus production and thereby decrease the stimulus for cough.

Massive Hemoptysis

Survival is so poor in patients with massive hemoptysis that they may not want any kind of intervention to stop the bleeding; in such cases, maintenance of comfort alone becomes the priority. For those patients who want intervention to stop the bleeding, the initial priority is to maintain a patent airway, which usually requires endotracheal intubation. Management options include endobronchial tamponade of the segment, vasoactive drugs, iced saline lavage, neodymium/yttrium-aluminum-garnet (Nd/YAG) laser photocoagulation, electrocautery, bronchial artery embolization, and external-beam or endobronchial irradiation.

Nonpharmacologic Interventions

If cough is induced by a sensitive cough reflex, then patients should attempt to avoid the stimuli that produce this. They should stop or cut down on smoking and avoid smoky rooms, cold air, exercise, and pungent chemicals. If medication is causing the cough, it should be decreased or stopped if possible. If the cause is esophageal reflux, then elevation of the head of the bed may be tried. Adequate hydration, humidification of the air, and chest physiotherapy may help patients expectorate viscid sputum. Radiation therapy to enlarged nodes, endoscopically placed esophageal stents for tracheoesophageal fistulas, or injection of Teflon into a paralyzed vocal cord may improve cough.

Patient and Family Teaching

Education should include practical matters such as proper use of medications, avoidance of irritants, use of humidification, and ways to improve the effectiveness of cough. One such way is called "huffing." The person lies on his or her side, supports the abdomen with a pillow, blows out sharply three times, holds the breath, and then coughs. This technique seems to improve the effectiveness of a cough and helps to expel sputum.

If the patient is having hemoptysis and massive bleeding is a possibility, it is important to educate the family about this possibility, to prepare them psychologically, and to develop a treatment plan. Dark towels or blankets can help to minimize the visual impact of this traumatic event. Adequate medications should be immediately available to control any anxiety or distress that might occur. Family and staff require emotional support after such an event.

Summary

Chronic cough can be a disabling symptom for patients. If the underlying cause is unresponsive to treatment, then suppression of the cough is the major therapeutic goal.

References

1. Mahler DA. Understanding mechanisms and documenting plausibility of palliative interventions for dyspnea. *Curr Opin Support Palliat Care*. 2011;5:71–76.

2. Solano JP, Gomes B, Higginson IJ. A comparison of symptom prevalence in far advanced cancer, AIDS, heart disease, chronic obstructive pulmonary disease and renal disease. *J Pain Symptom Manage*. 2006;31:58–69.
3. Currow D, Smith J, Davidson PM, Newton PJ, Agar MR, Abernethy AP. Do the trajectories of dyspnea differ in prevalence and intensity by diagnosis at the end of life? A Consecutive Cohort Study. *J Pain Symptom Manage*. 2010;39:680–690.
4. Lansing RW, Gracely RH, Banzett RB. The multiple dimensions of dyspnea: review and hypotheses. *Respir Physiol Neurobiol*. 2009;167:53–60.
5. Bausewein C, Farquhar M, Booth S, Gysels M, Higginson IJ. Measurement of breathlessness in advanced disease: a systematic review. *Respir Med*. 2006;101:399–410.
6. Woodcock AA, Gross ER, Gellert A, Shah S, Johnson M, Geddes DM. Effects of dihydrocodeine, alcohol, and caffeine on breathlessness and exercise tolerance in patients with chronic obstructive lung disease and normal blood gases. *N Engl J Med*. 1981;305:1611–1616.
7. Viola R, Kiteley C, Lloyd NS, Mackay JA, Wilson J, Wong RKS. The management of dyspnea in cancer patients: a systematic review. *Support Care Cancer*. 2008;16:329–337.
8. Ben-Aharon I, Gafter-Gvili A, Leibovici L, Stemmer SM. Interventions for alleviating cancer-related dyspnea: a systematic review. *J Clin Oncol*. 2008;26:2396–2404.
9. Clemens KE, Klaschik E. Symptomatic therapy of dyspnea with strong opioids and its effect on ventilation in palliative care patients. *J Pain Symptom Manage*. 2007;33:473–481.
10. Simon S, Higginson I, Booth S, Harding R, Bausewein C. Benzodiazepines for the relief of breathlessness in advanced malignant and non-malignant diseases in adults. The Cochrane Collaboration-Cochrane Pain, Palliative and Supportive Care Group. *Cochrane Database Syst Rev*. 2010(1):CD007354.
11. Navigante AH, Cerchietti LCA, Castro MA, Lutteral MA, Cabalar ME. Midazolam as adjunct therapy to morphine in the alleviation of severe dyspnea perception in patients with advanced cancer. *J Pain Symptom Manage*. 2006;31:38–47.
12. Cranston JM, Crockett A, Currow D. Oxygen therapy for dyspnoea in adults (Review). *Cochrane Library*. 2008;3:1–54.
13. Philip J, Gold M, Milner A, Di Iulio J, Miller B, Spruyt O. A randomized, double-blind, crossover trial of the effect of oxygen on dyspnea in patients with advanced cancer. *J Pain Symptom Manage*. 2006;32:541–550.
14. Abernethy AP, McDonald CF, Frith PA, et al. Effect of palliative oxygen versus room air in relief of breathlessness in patients with refractory dyspnoea: a double-blind, randomised controlled trial. *Lancet*. 2010;376:784–793.
15. Wildiers H, Menten J. Death rattle: prevalence, prevention and treatment. *J Pain Symptom Manage*. 2002;23:310–317.
16. Morita T, Hyodo I, Yoshima T, et al. Incidence and underlying etiologies of bronchial secretion in terminally ill cancer patients: a multicenter, prospective, observational study. *J Pain Symptom Manage*. 2004;27:533–539.
17. Wee BL, Coleman PG, Hillier R, Holgate ST. Death rattle: its impact on staff and volunteers in palliative care. *Palliat Med*. 2008;22:173–176.

18. Heisler M, Hamilton G, Chengalaram A, Koceja T, Gerkin R. Randomized double-blind trial of sublingual atropine vs. placebo for the management of death rattle. *J Pain Symptom Manage*. 2013;45:14–22.
19. Molassiotis A, Lowe M, Ellis J, et al. The experience of cough in patients diagnosed with lung cancer. *Support Care Cancer*. 2011;19:1997–2004.
20. Young EC, Smith JA. Pharmacologic therapy for cough. *Curr Opin Pharmacol*. 2011;11:224–230.

Chapter 3

Urgent Syndromes at the End of Life

Barton T. Bobb

Hallmarks of palliative care are skilled assessment and rapid evaluation and management of symptoms that negatively affect patient and family quality of life. This chapter addresses syndromes that unless recognized and treated promptly will cause unnecessary suffering for the patient and family at the end of life:

- Superior vena cava obstruction
- Pleural effusion
- Pericardial effusion
- Hemoptysis
- Spinal cord compression
- Hypercalcemia

Superior Vena Cava Obstruction

Definition

Superior vena cava obstruction (SVCO) is a disorder produced by obstruction of blood flow in the superior vena cava, which results in impairment of blood flow through the superior vena cava into the right atrium. Severity of the syndrome depends on rapidity of onset, location of the obstruction, and whether the obstruction is partial or complete. Obstruction may occur acutely or gradually, and symptoms may be severe and debilitating.[1]

Epidemiology

The patient most likely to experience SVCO is a 50- to 70-year-old man with a primary or metastatic tumor of the mediastinum. More than 90% of SVCO cases have been due to cancer, most commonly endobronchial tumors.[1] The percentage of SVCO cases due to nonmalignant causes is rising, primarily because of the higher use of intravascular devices. The prognosis of patients with SVCO strongly correlates with the prognosis of the underlying disease.

Two types of obstruction may cause SVCO: intrinsic obstruction and extrinsic obstruction.[1] Intrinsic obstruction is usually caused by primary tracheal malignancies that invade the airway epithelium, that is, squamous cell carcinoma and adenoid cystic carcinoma, as well as other benign and malignant tumors. Extrinsic obstruction occurs when airways are surrounded and compressed by external tumors or enlarged lymph nodes, that is, lymphoma and locally advanced thyroid, lung, or esophageal cancers. Obstruction may be caused by a tumor arising in the right main or upper lobe bronchus or by large-volume lymphadenopathy in the right paratracheal or precarinal lymph node chains.

Thrombosis of the superior vena cava (SVC) is also associated with insertion of indwelling catheters and central venous access devices, which are thought to damage the intima of vessels. Both adults and children may experience thrombosis of the SVC. More than compression or tumor, thrombosis is likely to cause acute and complete obstruction of the SVC. Cancer patients are also at greater risk for experiencing hypercoagulopathies, which increase the risk for experiencing thrombosis and SVCO. Other, less common nonmalignant causes associated with SVCO are mediastinal fibrosis from histoplasmosis and iatrogenic complications from cardiovascular surgery.[2]

Signs and Symptoms

The onset of symptoms is often insidious. Patients may report subtle signs that include venous engorgement in the morning hours after awakening from sleep, difficulty removing rings from fingers, and an increase in symptoms when bending forward or stooping, all of which may not be noticed initially.[1] The most common symptom of the syndrome is dyspnea. Swelling of the neck and face is seen in 50% of patients. Other common symptoms are cough (54%), arm swelling (18%), chest pain (15%), and dysphagia (9%).[2] Physical findings include venous distention of the neck (66%), venous distention of the chest wall (54%), facial edema (46%), plethora, a very ruddy facial complexion (19%), and cyanosis (19%). Patients may experience tachypnea, hoarseness, nasal stuffiness, periorbital edema, redness and edema of the conjunctivae, and, rarely, paralyzed vocal cord.[1,2]

In severe or rapid cases, when collateral circulation has not yet made accommodation for increased blood flow, symptoms may be immediately life threatening. Patients may experience orthopnea, stridor, respiratory distress, headache, visual disturbances, dizziness, syncope, lethargy, and irritability. As the condition further progresses, significant mental status changes occur, including stupor, coma, seizures, and, ultimately, death.

Diagnostic Procedures

Plain chest radiography is the least invasive diagnostic modality.[2] Computed tomography (CT) is the most widely available and used modality to elucidate the location, extent of obstruction or stenosis, presence and extent of thrombus formation, and status of collateral circulation. Magnetic resonance imaging (MRI) is another diagnostic tool that can confirm the diagnosis of SVC and distinguish between tumor mass and thrombosis.

Medical Management

Chemotherapy or mediastinal radiation therapy may be very effective as initial treatment for patients who have small cell lung cancer and SVCO at first presentation, as well as in those with recurrent or persistent disease. Radiation therapy is used in patients who have been previously treated with chemotherapy. However, because of side effects, large fractions should be avoided. When comparing the modalities used to treat SVCO, including chemotherapy alone, chemotherapy and radiation therapy, and radiation therapy alone, none has proved superior. Adverse prognostic indicators are dysphagia, hoarseness, and stridor.

Superior Vena Cava Stenting

Patients with severe symptoms are often best treated initially by SVC stenting, especially if a tissue diagnosis has not been made yet. However, the decision should be made on a case-by-case basis because many patients with lung cancer respond quickly to radiation or chemotherapy.[1] Although there are no controlled studies comparing radiation therapy with SVC stenting, several reviews and nonrandomized studies indicate that this procedure can relieve edema, promote improved superficial collateral vein drainage, and improve neurologic impairment. It can also relieve dyspnea, provide greater relief of obstruction, create few or minor complications, and allow for the full use of chemotherapy and radiation therapy, thus providing more rapid relief in a higher proportion of patients.[3] Complications associated with SVC stenting procedures include bleeding due to anticoagulation, arrhythmia, septic episodes, thrombosis, fibrosis, and migration of the stent.

Thrombolytic Therapies

Thrombolytic therapy has often been successful in the lysing of SVC thrombi.[1,2] Another alternative, percutaneous angioplasty with or without thrombolytics, may open SVC obstructions. Documented thrombi may be treated with tissue plasminogen activators.

Drug Therapy

Steroids have been one of the standard therapies for treatment of SVCO, despite the lack of research-based evidence to support their use. Prednisone and methylprednisolone have both been used to reduce inflammation in the treatment of SVCO, but the typical regimen is generally 4 mg of dexamethasone every 6 hours.[2] Diuretics may be given to promote diuresis, thus decreasing venous return to the heart, which reduces pressure in the SVC. However, caution must be exercised to avoid dehydration.

Nursing Management

The primary nursing goals are to identify patients at risk for developing SVC syndrome, to recognize the syndrome if it does occur, and to relieve dyspnea and other symptoms. Reduction of anxiety is another important nursing goal. The patient and family may experience significant distress not only because of physical symptoms experienced but also because of an altered physical appearance, including a ruddy, swollen, distorted face and neck.

The nurse monitors the patient for side effects of treatment and provides symptom management. For example, if the patient is receiving radiation therapy, the nurse should be alert for signs of dyspnea (which may indicate presence of tracheal edema), pneumonitis, dysphagia, pharyngitis, esophagitis, leukopenia, anemia, skin changes, and fatigue. If the patient is receiving chemotherapy, the nurse should be alert for signs of stomatitis, nausea and vomiting, fatigue, leukopenia, anemia, and thrombocytopenia. If the patient is receiving steroid therapy, the nurse should educate the patient and family about the potential for developing proximal muscle weakness, mood swings, insomnia, oral candida, and hyperglycemia. Aspects of palliative nursing care that are always of primary importance are early recognition and management of symptoms, educating the patient and family about these symptoms and what to report, and providing reassurance that these symptoms, if they occur, will be controlled.

Pleural Effusion

Definition

Pleural effusion is defined as a disparity between secretion and absorption of fluid in the pleural space secondary to increased secretion, impaired absorption, or both, resulting in excessive fluid collection.[4]

Epidemiology

Parapneumonic disease is the most common cause of pleural effusions, followed by malignant disease. Breast, ovarian, and lung cancer plus lymphomas account for most malignant pleural effusions (MPEs), followed by ovarian cancer and gastric cancer, in order of descending frequency.[4] Almost half of patients with metastatic disease will experience a pleural effusion sometime during the course of their disease. Pleural effusions can occur in hospitalized HIV patients, with the three leading causes being parapneumonic infection, pulmonary Kaposi's sarcoma, and tuberculosis.

Unfortunately, the presence of malignant pleural effusion is usually associated with widespread disease and poor clinical prognosis, particularly in patients with malignancy or AIDS. The overall mean survival for cancer patients who have MPE is 4 to 12 months.[5] Nearly all patients who have MPE are appropriate candidates for hospice care.

Diagnostic Procedures

A chest radiograph will usually establish the presence of the pleural effusion and should also differentiate the presence of free versus loculated pleural fluid. CT can show pleural or lung masses, adenopathy, pulmonary abnormalities such as infiltrates or atelectasis, or distant disease. Chest ultrasound may differentiate between pleural fluid and pleural-thickening disease.[4] In some cases, after evidence of the effusion has been established and obvious nonmalignant causes have been ruled out, a diagnostic thoracentesis may be helpful in establishing the diagnosis. Ultrasound guidance can avoid problems associated with performing "blind" thoracentesis.

Signs and Symptoms

Dyspnea is the most common symptom of pleural effusion and occurs in about 75% of patients.[4] Its onset may be insidious or abrupt and depends on how rapidly the fluid accumulates. It is almost always related to collapse of the lung from the increase of pleural fluid pressure on the lung.

The patient's inability to expand the lung leads initially to complaints of exertional dyspnea. As the effusion increases in volume, resting dyspnea, orthopnea, and tachypnea develop. The patient may complain of a dry, non-productive cough and an aching pain or heaviness in the chest. Pain is often described as dull or pleuritic in character. Generalized systemic symptoms associated with advanced disease may also be present: malaise, anorexia, and fatigue.[4]

Physical examination reveals the presence of dullness to percussion of the affected hemithorax, decreased breath sounds, egophony, decreased vocal fremitus, whispered pectoriloquy, and decreased or no diaphragmatic excursion. A large effusion may cause mediastinal shift to the side of the effusion; tracheal deviation may be present. Cyanosis and plethora, a ruddy facial complexion that occurs with partial caval obstruction, may also be present.

Medical Management

Overall medical management of malignant pleural effusion depends on multiple factors, including the history of the primary tumor, prior patient history and response to therapy, extent of disease and overall medical condition, goals of care, and severity of symptom distress. In some cases, systemic therapy, hormonal therapy, or mediastinal radiation therapy may provide control of pleural effusions.[4] Symptomatic management with pharmacotherapy includes the use of opioids to manage pain and dyspnea, as well as anxiolytics to control concomitant anxiety.

If the patient is to have a chest tube placed or other invasive procedures to drain the fluid or to prevent fluid reaccumulation, the nurse must aggressively manage the patient's pain and anxiety. Educating the patient about what to expect, being present during the procedure, and medicating the patient preemptively are important aspects of palliative nursing care. Use of patient-controlled analgesia for pain management is appropriate. Unfortunately, pain assessment and management are frequently not recognized as a priority when patients undergo these procedures.

Thoracentesis Alone

Thoracentesis has been shown to relieve dyspnea associated with large pleural effusions. When thoracentesis is undertaken, relief of symptoms may rapidly occur, but fluid reaccumulates quickly, usually within 3 to 4 days. The decision to perform repeated thoracenteses should be tempered by the knowledge that risks include empyema, pneumothorax, trapped lung from inadequate drainage or loculated fluid, and the possibility of increasing malnutrition as a result of the removal of large amounts of protein-rich effusion fluid. Repeated thoracenteses rarely provide lasting control of malignant effusions. Instead of a second thoracentesis, a thoracostomy with pleurodesis should be considered. It can be used to reduce adhesions, draw off fluid, and initiate drainage, all at the same time.

Tube Thoracostomy and Pleurodesis

Palliative treatment, especially for those with a life expectancy of months rather than weeks, is best accomplished by performing closed-tube thoracoscopy, using imaging guidance with smaller bore tubes. The goal of this therapy is to drain the pleural cavity completely, expand the lung fully, and then instill the chemical agent into the pleural cavity. However, if there is a large effusion, only 1,000 to 1,500 mL should be drained initially.[4] Too-rapid drainage of a large volume of fluid can cause reexpansion pulmonary edema, and some patients have developed large hydropneumothoraces after rapid evacuation of fluid.[4] The thoracoscopy tube should then be clamped for 30 to 60 minutes. Approximately 1,000 mL can be drained every hour until the chest is completely empty, but a slow rate of drainage is recommended. The chest tube is then connected to a closed-drainage device. To prevent reexpansion pulmonary edema, water-seal drainage alone and intermittent tube clamping should be used to allow fluid to drain slowly.

Complications of chest tube placement include bleeding and development of pneumothorax, which occurs when fluid is rapidly removed in patients who have an underlying noncompliant lung. Patients who have chest tubes inserted should receive intrapleural bupivacaine or epidural and intravenous (IV) conscious sedation because the procedure can be moderately to severely painful.

Pleurodesis

Chest radiography is used to monitor the position of the tube after thoracostomy is completed. It is thought that tube irritation of the pleural cavity may encourage loculations, which can lessen the effectiveness of potential sclerosing agents. Current evidence indicates that it is not necessary to wait for drainage to fall below a certain level and that the sclerosing agent can be injected as soon as the lung is fully reexpanded. If the lung fails to expand and there is no evidence of obstruction or noncompliant lung, additional chest tube placement may be considered. Fibrinolysis with urokinase or streptokinase may improve drainage in cases in which fluid is still present or is thick or gelatinous. Intrapleural instillation of urokinase 100,000 units in 100-mL 0.9% saline can be attempted and the chest tube clamped for 6 hours, with suction then being resumed for 24 hours. After the pleural fluid has been drained and the lung is fully expanded, pleurodesis may be initiated. This can usually take place the day after chest tube insertion.

The purpose of pleurodesis is to administer agents that cause inflammation and subsequent fibrosis into the pleural cavity to produce long-term adhesion of the visceral and parietal pleural surfaces. The goal of this procedure is to prevent reaccumulation of pleural fluid. Various sclerosing agents are used to treat MPE. They include bleomycin, doxycycline, and sterilized asbestos-free talc. There is some research indicating that talc should be the agent of choice based on its success rate in preventing recurrence and its overall effectiveness.

Pleuroperitoneal Shunt

Pleuroperitoneal shunt is useful for patients who have refractory MPE despite sclerotherapy. Two catheters are connected by a pump to a chamber between the pleural cavity and the peritoneal cavity. Manually pushing the pumping chamber moves fluid from the pleural cavity to the peritoneal cavity. Releasing the compression moves the fluid from the pleural cavity into the chamber.

The major advantage of this device is that it can be used on an outpatient basis and allows the patient to remain at home. Its disadvantages include obstruction risk, infection, and tumor seeding; general anesthesia is needed for placement, and the device requires motivation and ability on the part of the patient to operate it. Most patients with advanced disease are unable to physically overcome the positive peritoneal pressure required to pump the device. Pumping is required hundreds of times a day, and therefore this device is not likely to be useful in those who are close to death.

Pleurectomy

Surgical stripping of the parietal pleura, with or without lung decortication (if the underlying lung is trapped), is effective, but it has a high complication rate and should be reserved for patients who have a reasonable life expectancy and physical reserve to withstand surgery.[4] Video-assisted thoracoscopy (VATS) and pleurectomy have been performed successfully in small, selected groups of patients. However, they are likely to be an inappropriate choice in the palliative care patient at end of life.

Indwelling Pleural Catheters

Indwelling pleural catheters can be placed under local anesthesia.[4] Patients who meet criteria for ambulatory therapy—that is, those with symptomatic, unilateral effusions and a reasonable performance status—may benefit from this therapy. It has been suggested that tunneled pleural catheters may permit long-term drainage and control of MPE in more than 80% to 90% of patients.[4] These catheters can be used to treat trapped lungs and large locules.

Small-bore tubes attached to gravity drainage bags or vacuum drainage have been reported to be successful on an outpatient basis. Rare complications include tumor seeding, obstruction, infection, cellulitis of tract site, and pain during drainage. If spontaneous pleurodesis does not occur, then continuing drainage may present management challenges. This treatment offers the potential for better quality of life and reduction in overall healthcare costs.

Subcutaneous Access Ports

In this procedure a fenestrated catheter is placed in the pleural cavity. It can be accessed for repeated drainage without risk for pneumothorax or hemothorax.[4] Complications include occlusion, kinking, and wound infection.

Nursing Management

Dyspnea and anxiety are primary symptoms experienced by the patient who has a pleural effusion. When invasive diagnostic procedures are being considered, these choices should be guided by the stage of disease, prognosis, the risk-to-benefit ratio of tests or interventions, pain management considerations, and the desires of the patient and family. The nurse can educate the patient and family about each procedure, including its purpose, how it is carried out, how pain will be addressed, and possible side effects or complications that may occur. This not only allows for informed consent but also may help to reduce anxiety and thus decrease dyspnea. A variety of nonpharmacologic techniques can relieve the patient's dyspnea and pain and can be used in combination with opioids and anxiolytics, as well as concurrently with medical treatment. These approaches include positioning the patient for comfort, using relaxation techniques, and providing oxygenation as appropriate. Aggressive pain assessment and monitoring are particularly important for patients who receive invasive procedures.

Pericardial Effusion

Definition

A pericardial effusion is defined as an abnormal accumulation of fluid or tumor in the pericardial sac.[6] Pericardial effusions can lead to life-threatening sequelae. They can be caused by malignancies and their treatment and by nonmalignant conditions. Pericardial effusions can lead to cardiac tamponade, which, if not treated, will cause cardiovascular collapse and death.

Epidemiology

Malignant disease is the most common cause of pericardial effusions. Pericardial effusion is most commonly associated with lung and breast cancer, leukemia, and lymphoma. Metastatic spread or local extension from esophageal tumors and from sarcomas, melanomas, and liver, gastric, and pancreatic cancers can also occur. Nonmalignant causes of pericardial effusions include pericarditis, congestive heart failure, uremia, myocardial infarction, and autoimmune disease, such as systemic lupus erythematosus. Other causes are infections, fungi, virus, tuberculosis, hypothyroidism, renal and hepatic failure, hypoalbuminemia, chest trauma, aneurysm, and complications of angiographic and central venous catheter procedures. Cancer treatment—related causes of pericardial effusion include radiation therapy to the mediastinal area of more than 4,000 cGy and anthracycline-based chemotherapies, such as doxorubicin.

Signs and Symptoms

Pericardial tamponade that results from metastatic disease has a gradual onset that may be chronic and insidious.[6] Vague symptoms may be reported. Early in the decompensation process it may be difficult to differentiate symptoms of cardiac dysfunction from the effects seen in advancing cancer. The severity of symptoms is related to volume of the effusion, rate of accumulation, and the patient's underlying cardiac function. Generally, rapid accumulation of fluid is associated with more severe cardiac tamponade. The most powerful predictor of the development of cardiac tamponade is the size of the pericardial effusion.

Dyspnea is the most common presenting symptom. The patient may complain of the inability to catch his or her breath, which progresses from dyspnea on exertion to dyspnea at rest. In advanced stages, the individual may be able to speak only one word at a time. Chest heaviness, cough, and weakness are also symptoms. Pressure on adjacent structures, that is, the esophagus, trachea, and lung, may increase.

Tachycardia occurs as a response to decrease in cardiac output. A narrowing pulse pressure (difference between systolic and diastolic blood pressure) may be seen when blood backs up in the venous system, causing the systolic blood pressure to decrease and the diastolic blood pressure to increase. Compression of the mediastinal nerves may lead to cough, dysphagia, hoarseness, or hiccups. Increased venous pressure in the chest may lead to gastrointestinal (GI) complaints, such as nausea. Retrosternal chest pain that increases when the patient is supine and decreases when the patient is leaning forward may occur but is often not present. Engorged neck veins, hepatomegaly, edema, and increased diastolic blood pressure are late signs of effusion. Anxiety, confusion, restlessness, dizziness, lightheadedness, and agitation related to hypoxemia may be present as the process progresses. Poor cardiac output will lead to complaints of fatigue and weakness.

As the effusion increases and the heart begins to fail, symptoms worsen, and dyspnea and orthopnea progress. Increasing venous congestion leads to peripheral edema. As cerebral perfusion worsens and hypoxemia increases, confusion increases. Ultimately, there is cardiovascular collapse, anuria, and decreased tissue perfusion, which cause obtundation, coma, and death. Patients with chronic symptomatic pericardial effusions often exhibit tachycardia, jugular venous distention, hepatomegaly, and peripheral edema.

When examining the patient, one should listen for early signs of cardiac tamponade:

- Muffled heart sounds, perhaps a positional pericardial friction rub, and weak apical pulse
- Presence of a compensatory tachycardia
- Abdominal venous congestion and possible peripheral edema
- Fever

The signs and symptoms of pericardial effusion and cardiac tamponade may be mistaken for those of other pulmonary complications or pleural effusions. Many cancer patients have both pleural and pericardial effusions. Unfortunately, symptoms of cardiac tamponade may be the first indication of the presence of pericardial effusion.

The triad of hypotension, increased jugular venous pressure, and quiet heart sounds that are diagnostic for pericardial effusion occurs in less than one third of patients. Presence of clear lung fields can help the clinician differentiate between pericardial effusion and congestive heart failure. Pulsus paradoxus is a cardinal sign of cardiac tamponade. Pulsus paradoxus is a fall in systolic blood pressure of greater than 10 mm Hg with inspiration. Normally, blood pressure lowers on inspiration, but when the heart is compressed it receives even less blood flow. The resulting lowered volume and output result in a greater decrease in blood pressure. Hepatojugular reflux is a late sign of cardiac tamponade.

Late in the process of deterioration, diaphoresis and cyanosis are also present. The patient develops increasing ascites, hepatomegaly, peripheral edema, and central venous pressure. Decreased renal flow progresses to anuria. Further impairment in tissue perfusion leads to loss of consciousness, obtundation, coma, and death.

Diagnostic Procedures

Initially, a standard chest radiograph is likely to show a change in the size or contour of the heart and clear lung fields. Chest radiography can also demonstrate mediastinal widening or hilar adenopathy. This diagnostic tool is cost-effective, minimally invasive, and readily available and may detect tamponade before the patient becomes symptomatic. However, when used alone, it is not specific enough to diagnose pericardial effusions and does not indicate the level of heart decompensation. Two-dimensional echocardiogram is the most sensitive and precise test to determine whether pericardial effusion or cardiac tamponade is present. It can be used at the bedside and is noninvasive.

Other tests, including MRI and CT, can be used to detect effusions, pericardial masses and thickening, and cardiac tamponade. However, these tests do not indicate how well the heart is functioning, and they have limited use because of safety and comfort concerns in very ill patients. If echocardiography is not available, a cardiac catheterization, which will detect depressed cardiac output and pressure levels in all four chambers of the heart, may be considered on a case-by-case basis.

Medical Management

Options for medical management include pericardiocentesis with or without catheter drainage, pericardial sclerosis, percutaneous balloon pericardiotomy, pericardiectomy, pericardioperitoneal shunt, tunneled pericardial catheters, radiation therapy and chemotherapy, and aggressive symptom management without invasive procedures.

Pericardiocentesis

The most simple, safe, and effective (97%) treatment is echocardiography-guided pericardiocentesis. The procedure can be performed emergently at the bedside, blindly, or with electrocardiogram guidance, but it should not be attempted in this manner except in extreme emergencies. Adverse complications of the blind procedure include myocardial laceration, myocardial "stunning," arrhythmias, pneumothorax, abscess, and infection.

Pericardial Sclerosis

Patients who experience pericardial tamponade face a 50% rate of recurrence when the underlying disease is not effectively treatable. Pericardial sclerosis is defined as the instilling of chemicals through an indwelling catheter into the pericardial sac for the purpose of causing inflammation and fibrosis, to prevent further fluid reaccumulation. Doxycycline and bleomycin are the most common drugs instilled into the pericardial space. A common side effect of sclerosing therapy is severe retrosternal chest pain, especially with talc administration, and sometimes with bleomycin therapy. A preemptive pain management plan is essential for the well-being of the patient. Arrhythmias, catheter occlusion, and transient fever without associated bacteremia are also associated complications, primarily of talc and bleomycin therapy. A serious discussion of risks, benefits, side effects of the therapy, and its impact on quality of life should take place in the context of end-of-life decision making.

Percutaneous Balloon Pericardiotomy

Percutaneous balloon pericardiotomy is a safe, nonsurgical method that can be used to relieve the symptoms of chronic recurrent pericardial effusions.[6] It is performed in a cardiac catheterization laboratory under fluoroscopic guidance using IV conscious sedation and local anesthesia. A guidewire is inserted into the pericardial space, and a small pigtail catheter is inserted over the wire. The wire is removed, and some pericardial fluid is withdrawn. Next, the pigtail catheter is removed and replaced with a balloon-dilating catheter that is advanced into the pericardial space and inflated. A pericardial drainage catheter is left in place and is removed when there is less than 100 mL of drainage daily. Patients have reported experiencing severe pain during and after this procedure. A plan for aggressive pain management must be in place before this procedure and rapidly implemented if pain occurs. Fever and pneumothorax are the most common complications. Pleural effusion has also been associated with the procedure. It is suggested that percutaneous balloon pericardiotomy can be used in place of surgical drainage in patients with malignancy and a short life expectancy.

Surgical Pericardiectomy

Another option is to surgically create a pericardial "window" (partial pericardiectomy), a small opening in the pericardium, and suture it to the lung. This allows pericardial fluid to drain out of the pericardial cavity, especially loculated effusions. When other procedures fail and the patient is expected to have long-term survival and good quality of life, partial or complete pericardiectomy may be considered.

Video-Assisted Thoracoscopic Surgery

VATS, a minimally invasive procedure, can be used to manage chronic pericardial effusions. In this case, a thoracoscope is introduced into the left or right chest, and a pericardial window is performed under thoracoscopic vision.[7] The pleura and pericardium can be visualized, tissue diagnosis can be obtained, and loculated effusions can be drained.

Radiation Therapy and Chemotherapy

In some cases, radiation therapy can be used to treat chronic effusions after the pericardial effusion has been drained and when tamponade is not present. It can be effective in radiosensitive tumors such as leukemia and lymphomas but is less so in solid tumors. Systemic chemotherapy can be considered if the malignancy is chemotherapy sensitive.

Nursing Management

The priority goals in managing this condition are to provide comfort, to promote pain relief, and to reduce anxiety. The nurse should know both early and late signs of cardiac tamponade. Early recognition of these signs and their implications is most important because early intervention may prevent life-threatening sequelae. Aggressive symptom management includes the administration of opioids and anxiolytics to reduce pain and anxiety. If invasive cardiac procedures are carried out in an emergency at the bedside, the nurse should be present to provide support to the patient and family, to control pain and anxiety, and to monitor vital signs as indicated.

Hemoptysis

Definition

Hemoptysis is defined as blood that is expectorated from the lower respiratory tract. Hemoptysis can be classified according to the amount of blood expectorated: (1) mild—less than 15 to 20 mL in a 24-hour period; (2) moderate—greater than 15 to 20 mL but less than 200 mL in a 24-hour period; and (3) massive—greater than 200 to 600 mL in a 24-hour period.[8] The primary risk to the patient is asphyxiation from blood clot formation obstructing the airway, rather than from exsanguination. Massive hemoptysis carries a high mortality rate if not treated.

Epidemiology

Tuberculosis is the most common worldwide cause of hemoptysis.[8] The most common causes of hemoptysis in the United States are bronchitis, bronchiectasis, and bronchogenic carcinoma.[8] Other nonmalignant causes of hemoptysis are lung abscess, sarcoidosis, mycobacterium invasion, emphysema, fungal diseases, and AIDS. There is no underlying cause found in 15% to 30% of hemoptic episodes.[8]

Diagnostic Procedures

Flexible fiberoptic bronchoscopy is initially the quickest and surest way to visualize the source of bleeding in the upper lung lobes and to localize it in the lower respiratory tract.[8] This procedure can be done at the bedside without putting the patient under general anesthesia, and it can also visualize distal airways. If there is brisk bleeding, the rigid bronchoscope can suction more efficiently, remove clots and foreign bodies, allow for better airway control, and be used to obtain material for diagnostic purposes. Bronchoscopy should not be undertaken if there is evidence of pulmonary embolism, pneumonia, or bronchitis or when the patient's condition is so poor or unstable that no further intervention would be undertaken no matter what the results.

If treatment is to be initiated, the combination of bronchoscopy and high-resolution CT can identify the cause of hemoptysis in most patients. It is also quick, noninvasive, and less costly than other modalities. If pulmonary embolism is suspected and therapy is to be initiated, a ventilation-perfusion scan may be warranted.[8]

Signs and Symptoms

Respiratory complaints that raise suspicion of bleeding into the lungs may include cough, dyspnea, wheezing, chest pain, sputum expectoration, and systemic clues, such as fever, night sweats, and weight loss. Clues to nasopharyngeal bleeding as the possible source include frequent nosebleeds, throat pain, tongue or mouth lesions, dysphonia, and hoarseness. Clues to GI bleeding as the possible source include the presence of dyspepsia, heartburn, or dysphagia. "Coffee grounds" vomitus or blood in vomitus does not rule out hemoptysis because blood from respiratory sources can be swallowed. Patients and family members should be asked to describe the color of the blood and should be asked about any changes in color and pattern of bleeding in vomitus and stool.

During an active bleeding episode, a focused examination should be performed as quickly as possible. If possible, the nasopharynx, larynx, and upper airways should be thoroughly visually examined to rule out an upper airway source of bleeding. If bleeding is brisk and views are obstructed, examination may best be accomplished with bronchoscopy. The patient may be coughing or vomiting blood and may be short of breath. If possible, sputum, blood, and vomitus should be examined. Some patients may not yet have a diagnosis of malignancy. In these cases one should note clubbing of fingernails and presence of cervical or supraclavicular adenopathy. This may indicate the presence of a malignancy.

Massive bleeding may take place in the lung without the presence of hemoptysis, so listening to lung sounds is very important. Auscultation of the lungs may reveal localized wheezing, an indication of possible airway obstruction. Fine diffuse rales and asymmetrical chest excursion may indicate the presence of an infectious or consolidative process. If petechiae and ecchymosis are present, then there should be strong suspicion that a bleeding diathesis is present.

Medical Management

If the episode of bleeding is severe and the goal is active treatment or prolongation of life, then the primary focus is to maintain an adequate airway. This will usually require endotracheal intubation, which may have to be performed immediately at the bedside, and oxygenation. If bleeding can be localized and controlled quickly, a short period of intubation may be considered if it will allow for improved quality of life. Specific methods of treatment include radiation therapy, laser coagulation therapy, bronchial arterial embolization, endobronchial balloon tamponade, epinephrine injection, iced saline lavage, and, in very rare cases, surgical resection.

Radiation Therapy

External-beam radiation therapy can stop hemoptysis in more than 80% of cases, especially in those patients who have unresectable lung cancers. The goal is to provide therapy in the shortest time period possible, at the lowest dose to achieve symptom control while minimizing side effects. Endobronchial brachytherapy has been effective in some patients who have failed previous external-beam radiation attempts.

Endobronchial Tamponade

In this procedure, flexible bronchoscopy is used to find the bleeding site after the site has been lavaged with iced saline. A balloon catheter attached to the tip of the bronchoscope is placed on the site and is then inflated and left on the bleeding site for 24 to 48 hours.[9] This is not a uniformly successful procedure and should be considered a temporizing measure only.

Laser Coagulation Therapy

In the case of obstructing tracheal tumors, Nd-YAG photocoagulation may control bleeding from endobronchial lesions; however, highly vascular tumors are at risk for bleeding when exposed to laser therapy.

Bronchial Arterial Embolization

When an endoscopically visualized lung cancer is the source of bleeding, bronchial artery embolization is effective as a palliative intervention. Bronchial artery embolization, preceded by bronchoscopy, involves injecting a variety of agents angiographically into the bronchial artery to stop blood flow.

Endobronchial Epinephrine Injections

A 1:10,000 epinephrine solution may be instilled on visualized lesions to constrict veins and reduce bleeding. Vasopressin and chlorpromazine have also been used in this procedure, which is performed in patients who are not candidates for surgery and when bronchial artery embolization is not available.

Iced Saline Lavage

Iced saline solution lavage has been used as a temporary nonstandard measure to provide improved visualization and localization of the bleeding site. It does not appear to improve outcomes.

Surgery

In rare cases, some patients who continue to have life-threatening hemorrhage after receiving other therapies may be considered as candidates for surgical intervention. Only those whose life expectancy, condition, ability to tolerate major surgery, and ability to maintain an airway should be considered. It is important to remember that most lung cancers are well advanced at diagnosis and that undertaking this procedure may not meet quality-of-life goals for those with short-term prognoses.

Nursing Management

When a decision has been made to forego aggressive treatment measures, then promotion of comfort for the patient is the primary goal. Death from massive hemoptysis is usually rapid, occurring within minutes. However, even when the family has been carefully "prepared" for this possibility and coached in a step-by-step manner in what to do, family members inevitably remain unprepared and distraught if a massive hemorrhage does occur, especially in the home without medical personnel around. Preemptive planning includes anxiolytics and opioids readily available in the home, a 24-hour palliative care number to call for immediate guidance and support, and dark-colored towels to reduce the visibility of blood and thus make it less overwhelming.

Spinal Cord Compression

Definition

Spinal cord compression (SCC) is compression of the thecal sac at the level of the spinal cord or cauda equina. Spinal cord injury may cause progressive and irreversible neurologic damage and requires immediate intervention to prevent disability. SCC in the presence of malignancy often carries a poor prognosis, with a median life expectancy of 3 to 6 months.[10] Prognostic factors for longer survival include only one site of cord compression, ability to ambulate before and after treatment, bone metastases only, and tumor that is responsive to radiation.[10]

Epidemiology

Compression of the spinal cord and cauda equina is a major cause of morbidity in patients with cancer. It occurs in approximately 5% to 10% of patients with malignant disease and is most commonly associated with metastatic disease from tumors of the breast, lung, and prostate. Less than 50% of patients will regain functional losses because of SCC.

Compression of the spine in 85% to 90% of cases is caused by direct hematologic extension of solid tumor cells into a vertebral body. A less common pathway is by direct extension of tumor from adjacent tissue through the intervertebral foramina. Tumor cells can also enter the epidural space directly by circulating in the cerebral spinal fluid. Paraneoplastic syndromes, leptomeningeal disease, and toxicity of chemotherapy drugs can cause spinal cord syndromes. Nonmalignant causes of SCC include benign tumors; degenerative, inflammatory, and infectious diseases that affect the spinal column; and trauma, herniated disks, osteoporosis, and other structural diseases.

Diagnostic Procedures

Plain spinal radiographs are an excellent screening tool and can determine the presence of tumor and the stability of the spine. They can identify lytic or blastic lesions in up to 85% of vertebral lesions. However, false-negative results can occur because of poor visualization, mild pathology, or poor interpretation. Epidural spread of tumor through the foramina might not always be visualized using plain radiographs. A bone scan may detect vertebral abnormalities when plain films are negative. MRI is the imaging choice for emergent SCC. It is noninvasive and does not require injection with contrast material. It has an advantage over CT because it can image the entire spine, thus detecting multiple areas of compression. Decisions about diagnostic testing will be tempered by a number of factors, including the potential for treatment, prognosis, patient's condition, and the patient's and family's wishes for treatment.

Signs and Symptoms

The presence of increasing back pain, worse on lying flat and improved on standing, with or without signs of bowel and bladder impairment, in a patient with a history of cancer should be presumed to be SCC until proved otherwise. Neurologic function before initiation of therapy is the single most important prognostic factor in SCC. Misdiagnosis of SCC has been attributed to poor history, inadequate examination, and insufficient diagnostic evaluation. Sensory changes occur in about half of patients at presentation. Sensory change without pain complaint is extremely rare.

A thorough history should pay special attention to the onset of pain; its location, intensity, duration, and quality; and what activities increase or decrease the pain. A history of sensory or motor weakness and autonomic dysfunction should be evaluated and should include onset and degree of weakness; heaviness or stiffness of limbs; difficulty walking; numbness in arms, hands, fingers, toes, and trunk; and change in temperature or touch. Specific questions about bowel, bladder, and sexual function should be asked directly because patients may not volunteer these symptoms, such as difficulty in passing urine or stool, incontinence of bowel or bladder, loss of sphincter control, and ability to obtain and maintain an erection. Constipation usually precedes urinary retention or incontinence.

Physical examination includes observation of the spine, muscles, extremities, and skin and palpation and gentle percussion of vertebrae. Spinal manipulation to elicit pain responses should be carried out cautiously because it may cause muscle spasm or further injury. Mental status, cranial nerves, motor function, reflexes, sensation, coordination, strength, and gait should be evaluated (when appropriate to the patient's status and closeness to death). Focused examination may include performing straight-leg raises until the patient feels pain, then dorsiflexing the foot. If this action increases pain down the back of the leg, this suggests that nerve root compression is present. Testing of reflexes will indicate the presence and impact of nerve root compression on motor ability. Cord compression may cause hyperactive deep-tendon reflexes, whereas nerve root compression may cause decreased deep-tendon reflexes. A positive Babinski sign and sustained ankle clonus indicate motor involvement.

Sensory function should be tested by assessing pain (sharp, dull), temperature (hot, cold), touch (light), vibration (tuning fork test), and position senses (fingers and toes). Examination may reveal a demarcated area of sensory loss and brisk or absent reflexes. The mapping of positive sensation can be used to pinpoint the level of SCC, usually one or two levels below the site of compression. Bladder percussion and digital rectal examination will elicit retention and laxity of sphincter control, a late sign of SCC.

Pain may be reported for weeks to months before any obvious neurologic dysfunction. Pain may be local initially (e.g., in the central back), then progress to a radicular pattern that follows a particular dermatome. Local pain may be caused by stretching of bone periosteum by tumor or vertebral collapse and is usually described by the patient as constant, dull, aching, and progressive in nature. Radicular pain is caused by pressure of tumor along the length of the nerve root. The patient who reports radicular pain will describe it as shooting, burning, or shocklike in nature and will state that it is worsened by movement, coughing, sneezing, straining, neck flexion, or lying down. A classic sign of cord compression is pain that is relieved by sitting up or standing and is worsened by lying flat. Also, if pain increases at night when the patient is lying down to sleep, one should be suspicious of SCC rather than degenerative or disk disease. Radicular pain is typically bilateral in thoracic lesions and is often described as a tight band around the chest or abdomen, but it may also be experienced in only part of one dermatome.

The sequence of neurologic symptoms usually progresses in the following manner: first there is pain, then motor weakness that progresses to sensory loss, then motor loss, and finally autonomic dysfunction. The patient will initially complain of heaviness or stiffness in the extremities, loss of coordination, and ataxia. Sensory complaints include paresthesias and numbness and loss of heat sensation. Dysfunction begins in the toes and ascends in a stocking-like pattern to the level of the lesion. Loss of proprioception, deep pressure, and vibration are late signs of sensory loss. When the cauda equina is affected, sensory loss is bilateral; the dermatome that follows the perianal area, posterior thigh, and lateral aspect of the leg is involved. Late signs of

SCC are motor loss and paralysis. Loss of sphincter control is associated with poor return to functionality.

Medical Management

The focus of management of SCC should be the relief of pain and preservation or restoration of neurologic function. Rapid intervention is required to prevent permanent loss of function and concomitant quality of life. The patient status (e.g., goals of care and closeness to death), rate of neurologic impairment, and prior radiation therapy experience are other factors to consider.[10] Corticosteroids, surgical decompression, radiation therapy, and adjuvant chemotherapy or hormonal therapy are the standard treatments for SCC.[11]

Corticosteroids

Corticosteroids decrease vasogenic edema and inflammation and thus relieve pain and neurologic symptoms, and may have some oncolytic effect on tumor. Dexamethasone is the preferred corticosteroid because it is less likely to promote systemic edema caused by other steroids or to cause cognitive and behavioral dysfunction, and it improves overall outcomes after specific therapy. There has been controversy about dosage and scheduling of dexamethasone therapy in the management of SCC. A recent Cochrane review examining interventions for metastatic extradural SCC was, however, unable to demonstrate any evidence-based differences in benefit from high-dose versus low-dose corticosteroids. The review did, however, conclude that the incidence of adverse side effects was greater with high-dose compared with low-dose steroid therapy.[11] One suggested approach would be to administer high-dose therapy for patients who are no longer ambulatory or have rapidly increasing motor deficits, and low-dose therapy for those patients who can walk and do not have significant or worsening motor deficits.

Currently, high-dose therapy regimens recommend administering a 100-mg IV bolus of dexamethasone, followed by 24 mg dexamethasone orally four times daily for 3 days, then tapering the dose over 10 days. High-dose therapy may increase analgesia but, as mentioned, can also increase side effects that are significant. These include GI bleeding, hyperglycemia, depression and psychosis, myopathy, osteoporosis, and acute adrenal insufficiency with abrupt withdrawal. Low-dose dexamethasone regimen recommends administering a 10-mg IV bolus of dexamethasone, followed by 4 mg IV four times daily for 3 days, then tapering the dose over 14 days. Rapid IV push of corticosteroids causes severe burning pain in the perineum, and the patient needs to be warned that this will occur but does not signify that anything is wrong.

Decompressive Surgery

The goals of surgery are to decompress neural structures, resect tumor if possible, establish local disease control, achieve spinal stability, restore the ability to ambulate, treat pain, and improve quality of life. Surgery for SCC has been used to (1) establish a diagnosis when tissue is required for histologic analysis; (2) halt rapidly deteriorating function; (3) achieve cure for primary malignancy; (4) treat those with previously irradiated radioresistant tumor and continuing symptomatic progressive loss of function; (5) rule out infection or hematoma; (6) alleviate respiratory paralysis caused by high cervical spinal cord lesions; and (7) decompress and stabilize spine structure.[12] Benefits and burden of surgery to the patient in a palliative care setting must be carefully weighed so that the patient and family can make an informed decision.

Radiation Therapy

Fractionated external-beam radiation therapy to the spine is given to inhibit tumor growth, restore and preserve neurologic function, treat pain, and improve quality of life. It has been the primary treatment for SCC. The standard treatment regimen is 30 Gy over the course of 10 fractions, but hypofractionation (e.g., 8 Gy once or 4 Gy over five fractions) maybe used in patients with limited expected survival.

Nursing Management

The goal of nursing management is to identify patients at high risk for cord compression, to educate the patient and family regarding signs and symptoms to report, to detect early signs of SCC, and to work as a member of the palliative care team in managing symptoms. In patients who have far-advanced disease, palliative care efforts focus on promoting comfort, relieving pain, and providing family support.

Hypercalcemia

Definition

Hypercalcemia is an excessive amount of ionized calcium in the blood. If hypercalcemia is left untreated, the patient may experience irreversible renal damage, coma, or death. Mortality from untreated hypercalcemia approaches 50%.

Epidemiology

About 10% to 20% of cancer patients will develop hypercalcemia at some time during their illness.[13] Carcinomas of the breast and lung, multiple myeloma, and squamous cell carcinomas of the head, neck, and esophagus are the most common malignancies associated with hypercalcemia. Primary hyperparathyroidism as a cause of hypercalcemia is more common in the ambulatory and asymptomatic population. Other conditions associated with hypercalcemia include lithium therapy, Addison's disease, Paget's disease, granulomatous disease, vitamin D intoxication, hyperthyroidism, vitamin A intoxication, and aluminum intoxication.

Diagnostic Tests and Procedures

The ionized calcium concentration is the most important laboratory test to use in the diagnostic workup for hypercalcemia. It is the most accurate indicator of the level of calcium in the blood. (There is only a fair correlation between the total serum calcium level and ionized calcium.) When ionized calcium cannot be used as a diagnostic tool, the total serum calcium value may be used, but it must be corrected for serum albumin. A rule of thumb is to add 0.8 for each 1 g/dL decrease in albumin below the normal range (3.7 to 5 g/dL).

Signs and Symptoms

Symptoms of hypercalcemia, their severity, and how quickly they appear will vary from patient to patient. The extent of metastatic bone disease is not associated with hypercalcemia levels. It is important to remember that patients, especially elderly and debilitated patients, may experience severe symptoms even when serum calcium is not extremely elevated. Symptoms of hypercalcemia, such as vomiting, nausea, anorexia, weakness, constipation, and impaired mental status, may be mistakenly attributed to the disease or effects of treatment. Factors that will influence patients' response to hypercalcemia include age, performance status, renal or hepatic failure, and sites of metastatic disease.

Patients with a corrected serum calcium level of less than 12 mg/dL who are asymptomatic can be considered to have mild hypercalcemia. Patients who have a serum calcium level between 12 and 14 mg/dL should be closely monitored and may require urgent intervention, depending on goals of care in the palliative setting. Patients with a calcium level greater than 14 mg/dL will require urgent treatment, again depending on goals of care in the palliative setting.[13]

The patient may report numerous symptoms that can mimic symptoms of advanced malignancy. These include GI symptoms of nausea, vomiting, anorexia, constipation, obstipation, and even complete ileus. Polydipsia and polyuria may also be present. Muscle weakness, fatigue, and difficulty climbing stairs or getting out of a car are musculoskeletal symptoms that can progress to profound weakness, hypotonia, and fracture. Neuropsychological symptoms can begin with confusion, personality change, restlessness, and mood alterations and can progress to slurred speech, psychotic behavior, stupor, and coma. These are also symptoms that must be evaluated. The patient may also complain of bone pain, although the precise mechanism of bone-pain hypercalcemia is unknown.

Early signs of delirium in the hypercalcemic patient are associated with multiple factors that include electrolyte imbalance, metabolic disturbance, and renal failure, among others. If recognized early, treatment of the condition can alleviate and possibly reverse the symptoms. Management of confusion includes both pharmacotherapy and a reassuring and calm environment.

Medical Management

Regardless of the goals of care, active treatment goals are to promote alleviation of distressing symptoms. All patients with hypercalcemia who are symptomatic warrant a trial of therapy. When the goal is to reverse the hypercalcemia, this is accomplished by replenishing depleted intravascular volume, promoting diuresis of calcium, shutting down osteoclast activity in the bone, inhibiting renal tubular reabsorption of calcium, and promoting patient mobilization to the extent it is possible.[13]

Hydration is the first step in treatment. The purpose of hydration is to increase urinary calcium excretion, which improves renal function. One to

2 liters of isotonic saline are administered over 1 to 4 hours, and the patient's fluid intake and urinary output are closely monitored. The rate of fluid administration depends on the clinical estimate of the extent of hydration, patient's cardiovascular function, and renal excretion capacity.

Electrolytes and other laboratory values are closely monitored in appropriate patients. These include serum calcium (ionized or corrected), potassium, magnesium, other electrolytes, and albumin and bicarbonate levels. Renal function tests, including blood urea nitrogen and creatinine, are monitored. In rare cases, dialysis may be considered. In most patients, cardiac effects of hypercalcemia are minimal and outcomes are not usually affected, so cardiac monitoring is not usually necessary.

Bisphosphonate Therapy

Most hypercalcemic patients are treated with bisphosphonate therapy. It is an effective therapy for a number of cancers.[14] Bisphosphonate therapy inhibits bone resorption by osteoclasts, thus reducing the amount of calcium released into the bloodstream. Several IV bisphosphonates and aminobisphosphonates are available for use in patients. Pamidronate, etidronate, risedronate sodium, ibandronate, and zoledronate are available in the United States.

Pamidronate has been the most frequently used bisphosphonate, but zoledronate is becoming more widely used in the outpatient setting because of its much more rapid infusion time (30 minutes versus 2 to 6 hours for pamidronate). Pamidronate is usually given as 60 to 90 mg IV approximately every 3 to 4 weeks. In general, there is a 60% response to a 60-mg dose and a 100% response to a 90-mg dose.[13] Zoledronate, usually given as 4 mg IV, has been shown to have a higher rate and duration of control of hypercalcemia compared with pamidronate.[13] Pamidronate, and especially zoledronate, can cause renal toxicity (thus making evaluation and continued monitoring of kidney function essential before and during administration). Bisphosphonates can cause osteonecrosis of the jaw, especially in patients with myeloma who have been treated with pamidronate and zoledronate for a long period of time and in patients with dental problems.[13]

Because hypercalcemia tends to recur, pamidronate or zoledronate must be given approximately every 4 weeks. Immediate side effects of pamidronate therapy include low-grade fever appearing within 48 hours of treatment, redness, induration, and swelling at the site of catheter. Hypomagnesia and hypocalcemia may also occur. Rapid administration of IV bisphosphonates can cause significant pain, and this practice should be avoided. Subcutaneous administration of clodronate has been found to be an efficient treatment for malignant hypercalcemia. This route may be particularly useful in hospital, home, and hospice settings and spares the patient discomfort and the costs associated with transportation and IV administration in the hospital environment.

Calcitonin

Calcitonin inhibits resorption of calcium and can rapidly restore normocalcemia, often within 2 to 4 hours of administration. It is much less effective than pamidronate. Its role in managing hypercalcemia is limited to short-term use, usually of only 2 to 3 days' duration. Side effects are usually mild and include nausea and vomiting, skin rashes, and flushing. Calcitonin can be an alternative for treatment in patients with kidney failure (in whom pamidronate and zoledronate are contraindicated).[13]

Gallium Nitrate and Plicamycin

Gallium nitrate is an effective bone resorptive agent. Its mechanism of action is unknown. Its main disadvantages are that it has potential to cause nephrotoxicity, and it must be given as a continuous IV infusion over 5 days.

Plicamycin is an antitumor antibiotic. Its mechanism is unknown. It has a hypocalcemic effect that occurs within 48 hours of administration and that lasts for 3 to 7 days, but it exhibits marrow, hepatic, and renal toxicities. Individual response variations make this drug unpredictable, and it must be administered repeatedly.

Corticosteroids

Corticosteroids have a limited role in the treatment of hypercalcemia.

Dialysis

The use of dialysis has been reserved for patients who have severe hypercalcemia, renal failure, or congestive heart failure and cannot be given saline hydration. The decision to offer this therapy is made on a case-by-case basis, but, in general, dialysis is not offered in the palliative care arena.

Nursing Management

Hypercalcemia can cause significantly painful and distressing symptoms, including bone pain, agitation and confusion, severe constipation, and delirium. Treatment of hypercalcemia can reduce pain and other symptoms, improve quality of life, and reduce hospitalizations. At the end of life, the promotion of comfort and management of symptoms are the primary goals of palliative nursing care. If hypercalcemia cannot be reversed or the patient decides that the burden of interventions is greater than the benefit, the patient should be given the option of discontinuing such treatment. Ongoing management of symptoms, including sedation if desired, must be guaranteed to the patient and family.

Conclusion

This chapter addressed a group of syndromes, which, unless recognized and treated promptly, will cause unnecessary suffering for the patient and family. Emphasis has been given to the epidemiology and basic pathophysiology of each syndrome and to diagnostic assessment. Providing this information, although by necessity limited in detail, enables the palliative care nurse to explain to the patient and family why particular symptoms are occurring and why a particular management approach is being suggested. Treatment advice and decisions are always couched within the framework of the following questions: "Is the underlying cause reversible or not?" "What is the benefit-to-burden ratio of the treatment and how does that fit with the patient's values and goals?" "What is the likely outcome if the syndrome is not treated?" "How will resultant symptoms be managed?" "Is palliative sedation available to a patient at end of life if desired?" "Will the site of care affect treatment decisions?"

References

1. Walji N, Chan AK, Peake DR. Common acute oncological emergencies: diagnosis, investigation and management. *Postgrad Med J*. 2008;84:418–427.
2. Yu JB, Wilson LD, Detterbeck FC. Superior vena cava syndrome: a proposed classification system and algorithm for management. *J Thorac Oncol*. 2008;3:811–814.
3. Hague J, Tippett R. Endovascular techniques in palliative care. *Clin Oncol*. 2010;22:771–780.
4. Heffner JE, Klein JS. Recent advances in the diagnosis and management of malignant pleural effusion. *Mayo Clin Proc*. 2008;83:235–250.
5. Burrows CM, Mathews WC, Colt HG. Predicting survival in patients with recurrent symptomatic malignant pleural effusions: an assessment of the prognostic values of physiologic, morphologic, and quality of life measures of extent of disease. *Chest*. 2000;117:73–78.
6. Nguyen DM, Schrump DS. Malignant pleural and pericardial effusions. In: DeVita V, Hellman S, Rosenberg S, eds. *Cancer Principles and Practice of Oncology*. 7th ed. Philadelphia: Lippincott Williams & Wilkins; 2005:2381–2392.
7. Gross JL, Younes RN, Deheinzelin D, et al. Surgical management of symptomatic management of pericardial effusion in the patient with solid malignancies. *Ann Surg Oncol*. 2006;13:1732–1738.
8. Corder R. Hemoptysis. *Emerg Med Clinics N Am*. 2003;21:421–435.
9. Brandes JC, Schmidt E, Yung R. Occlusive endobrachial stent placement as a novel management approach to massive hemoptysis from lung cancer. *J Thorac Oncol*. 2008;3:1071–1072.
10. Cole JS, Patchell RA. Metastatic epidural spinal cord compression. *Lancet Neurol*. 2008;7:459–466.
11. George R, Jeba J, Ramkumar G, et al. Interventions for the treatment of metastatic extradural spinal cord compression in adults. *Cochrane Database Syst Rev*. 2008;4:CD006716.
12. Akram H, Allibone J. Spinal surgery for palliation in malignant spinal cord compression. *Clin Oncol*. 2010;22:792–800.
13. Lumachi F, Brunello A, Roma A, Basso U. Medical treatment of malignancy-associated hypercalcemia. *Curr Med Chem*. 2008;15:415–421.
14. Wong MHF, Stockler MR, Pavlakis N. Bone agents for breast cancer. *Cochrane Database Syst Rev*. 2012;2:CD003474.

Chapter 4

Sedation for Refractory Symptoms

Patti Knight, Laura A. Espinosa, and Bonnie Freeman

In the United States, approximately 2.5 million people die each year, with more than 60% of deaths occurring in hospitals and long-term care facilities.[1] This is despite the fact that most people report a wish to die in their home. This disparity is alarming and underscores the public's concern about care for the dying. Most studies reveal that patients and their family members wanted to be involved in decision making and to be comfortable at the end of life with well-managed symptoms and care that does not exhaust life savings.

Oregon's Death With Dignity Act has been in effect since 1997. This Act allows terminally ill Oregonians to end their lives through the voluntary self-administration of medications prescribed by a physician for that purpose. Before the law was passed, opponents argued that good palliative and hospice care would largely replace the need for such a law. In the first 10 years after the law was passed, 341 patients chose to end their life under the protection of the Death With Dignity Act. The Oregon Department of Health Services (ODHS) is required to collect information about patients and physicians who participate in the process. The 2007 ODHS report states that 33% of participating patients mentioned concern about pain (up from 26% in past years) as one reason for seeking a prescription for lethal medications. ODHS also reports that 100% of patients mentioned loss of autonomy as the main reason for seeking a prescription, and 86% cited decreasing ability to participate in enjoyable activities, as well as loss of dignity, as highly significant in their decision. In 2008, the State of Washington passed a Death With Dignity Act modeled after the Oregon law.[2] Obviously, this is an issue with which patients and the public are concerned. With this in mind, both nurses and physicians need to develop skills in assessing why a particular patient is requesting a hastened death so that appropriate interventions can be initiated.

Palliative care providers are faced with the challenge of managing a multitude of complex symptoms in terminally ill patients. Although many of these symptoms respond to skilled palliative management, others can remain refractory to treatment.[3] Suffering at the end of life involves physical, psychological, social, and spiritual distress. In most situations, multidisciplinary palliative interventions provide effective comfort, but in some instances suffering becomes refractory and intolerable. In these circumstances, palliative sedation may be necessary.

Definitions: From Terminal Sedation to Palliative Sedation

Numerous efforts have been made to standardize a definition for *terminal* and to separate sedation at end of life from sedation used in other medical settings.[3] Terms used for sedation at end of life include "palliative sedation," "terminal sedation," "total sedation,"[1] "sedation for intractable symptoms," and "sedation for distress in the imminently dying." Palliative sedation has been termed "slow euthanasia," although this is not a widely accepted definition of palliative sedation because the intent of sedation at end of life is to relieve suffering and not to hasten death.

Palliative sedation is defined as the monitored use of medications to induce sedation as a means to control refractory and unendurable symptoms near the end of life. The intent is to control symptoms, not hasten death. The acceptance of the term "palliative sedation" over "terminal sedation" has evolved to emphasize the difference between management of refractory symptoms at end of life and euthanasia. Box 4.1 lists common terms used in relation to palliative sedation and terminal weaning.

The goal of palliative sedation is the relief of suffering and includes the concept of proportionality. Proportionality, in this setting, implies that the patient's consciousness is reduced just enough to relieve refractory suffering. Depending on the patient's situation, the level of sedation that is required may be light or deep. The endpoint that is sought is the relief of suffering. This range in the depth of sedation is based on the "intentional administration of sedative drugs in dosages and combinations as required to reduce the consciousness of a terminally ill patient as much as necessary to relieve one or more refractory symptoms."[4] This definition reflects proportionality and clearly separates out palliative sedation at end of life from euthanasia.

Frequency of Palliative Sedation

Because the definition of palliative sedation is so varied, it is difficult to determine how often palliative sedation at end of life occurs in practice. Estimates range from 10% to 52%, varying by definition and practice sites.[3,4]

Reasons for Palliative Sedation

Deep sedation is a usual and accepted standard of practice before surgery or an extremely painful or highly distressing procedure. However, sedation at end of life does not have the same level of acceptance. Common symptoms at the end of life include pain, dyspnea, delirium, nausea, and vomiting, as well as feelings of hopelessness, remorse, anxiety, and loss of meaning. Palliative sedation is most commonly used and accepted for the relief of refractory physical symptoms. Claessens and colleagues, in a literature review of palliative sedation, found that most practitioners listed physical symptoms as the reasons for sedation at

Box 4.1 Palliative Sedation Definitions

Existential suffering (sometimes referred to as terminal anguish): Refractory psychological symptoms.

Imminent death: Death that is expected to occur within hours to days based on the person's condition, disease progression, and symptom constellation.

Intent: The purpose or state of mind at the time of an action. Intent of the patient/proxy and healthcare provider is a critical issue in ethical decision making regarding palliative sedation. Relief of suffering, not hastening or causing death, is the intent of palliative sedation.

Palliative sedation: The monitored use of medications intended to provide relief of refractory symptoms by inducing varying degrees of unconsciousness, but not death, in terminally ill patients. Levels of sedations are as follows:

Mild (somnolence): The patient is awake with a lowered level of consciousness.

Intermediate (stupor): The patient is asleep but can be awakened to communicate briefly.

Deep (coma): The patient is unconscious and unresponsive.

Double effect: In terminal sedation, an act with more than one potential effect (one good and one bad) is ethical if (1) the intended end (relief of distressing symptoms) is a good one; (2) the bad effect (death) is foreseen but not intended; (3) the bad effect is not the means of bringing about the good effect (death is not what relieves the distress); and (4) the good effect outweighs the bad effect (in a dying patient, the risk for hastening death for the benefit of comfort is appropriate).

Refractory symptom: A symptom that cannot be adequately controlled in a tolerable time frame despite the aggressive use of usual therapies and that seems unlikely to be adequately controlled by further invasive or noninvasive therapies without excessive or intolerable acute or chronic side effects.

end of life, with a smaller number indicating existential suffering as the reason for sedation. The most common physical symptoms were delirium, dyspnea, and pain. The nonphysical symptoms were feelings of meaninglessness, being a burden, dependency, and death anxiety and the wish to control the timing and manner of death.[4] Fainsinger and associates, in a multicenter international study, found that 1% to 4% of terminally ill patients needed sedation for pain, 0% to 6% for nausea and vomiting, 0% to 13% for dyspnea, and 9% to 23% for delirium.[5] Multiple physical and psychological symptoms are common.

Various factors that may affect varying standards of practice for palliative sedation include the physician's philosophy of what constitutes a "good death," personal and professional experiences, religious beliefs, and level of fatigue or burnout. Although there is no consensus on the use of palliative sedation for existential suffering, literature suggests that its use in these circumstances may be increasing.[6] Ganzini and colleagues reviewed Oregon physicians' perceptions of reasons that patients requested a hastened death and found that avoidance of dependency on others and wanting to control the timing and manner of their death were frequently cited.[7] In the intensive care unit (ICU) setting, reasons for palliative sedation are related to both refractory symptom management and terminal weaning from a ventilator.

Medications and Monitoring

Drugs most commonly used for palliative sedation outside the ICU setting are benzodiazepines, neuroleptics, barbiturates, and anesthetics.[3] Midazolam is the most commonly used of these drugs. The drug and route chosen vary based on the route available, location of the patient, and cost, as well as the preference of the provider. Usually in inpatient settings the medications are given intravenously or subcutaneously and continuously. In general, the chosen medication is started at a low dose and titrated upward rapidly until the symptom is controlled and the patient does not evidence signs of distress.

Table 4.1 Management of Distressing Physical Symptoms

Symptom	Considerations Before Defining a Symptom as Refractory
Agitation and confusion	Discontinue all nonessential medications.
	Change required medications to ones less likely to cause delirium.
	Check for bladder distention and rectal impaction.
	Evaluate for undiagnosed or undertreated pain.
	Review role of hydration therapy.
	Consider evaluation and therapy for potentially reversible processes, such as hypoxia, hyponatremia, and hypercalcemia.
Pain	Maximize opioid, nonopioid, and adjuvant analgesics, including agent, route, and schedule.
	Consider other therapies, including invasive or neurosurgical procedures, environmental changes, wound care, physical therapy, and psychotherapy.
	Anticipate and aggressively manage analgesic side effects.
Shortness of breath	Provide oxygen therapy if appropriate.
	Maximize opioid and anxiolytic therapy.
	Review the role of temporizing therapy, including thoracentesis, stents, and respiratory therapy.
Muscle twitching	Differentiate from seizure activity.
	Remember the use of opioid rotation, clonidine, and benzodiazepines if muscle twitching is caused by high-dose opioids.

Source: Cowan JD, Palmer TW. Practical guide to palliative sedation. *Curr Oncol Rep.* 2002;4:242–249.

Classes of medications used and routes of administration are presented in Table 4.1.[8]

Dose ranges are highly variable and determined by the patient's weight, renal and hepatic function, state of hydration, concurrent medication use, and other variables. The right dose is the dose that results in the patient resting comfortably without showing evidence of distress. It is recommended that doses be started low and titrated at approximately 30% an hour until sedation is achieved and the desired Richmond Agitation-Sedation Scale (RASS) level is reached[9] (Table 4.2).

The type of medication that can be administered by nurses may be influenced by state regulatory rules. The drugs used for refractory symptoms in the ICU include opiates, benzodiazepines, neuroleptics, and anesthetics.[10] These drugs can be continually infused and titrated until the patient appears comfortable. Morphine or other opioids are used to provide analgesia and reduce dyspnea. Propofol is a general anesthetic but can be used at sedative doses for ICU patients. Propofol is a good choice because of its rapid onset and rapid offset. Haloperidol is used in the treatment of delirium and can be combined with opiates and sedative agents to manage acute agitation or to protect against delirium in vulnerable patients. The drugs of choice for deep sedation are usually classified as anesthesia medications and therefore can only be used in monitored settings in most circumstances.

Assessment Tools to Measure Sedation and Agitation

Assessment tools to measure sedation and agitation are important in assessing and managing levels of consciousness in patients undergoing palliative

Table 4.2 Medications Used for Palliative Sedation

Medication	Dose and Route	Comments
Benzodiazepines Midazolam	Loading dose of 0.5–5.0 mg, followed by 0.5–10 mg/h continuously infused IV or SQ	Monitor for paradoxical agitation with all benzodiazepines
Lorazepam	0.5–5.0 mg every 1–2 h PO, SL, or IV	—
Neuroleptics Haloperidol	Loading dose of 0.5–5.0 mg PO, SL, SC, or IV, followed by an IV bolus of 1–5 mg every 4 h or 1–5 mg/h continuously infused IV or SQ	Monitor for extrapyramidal side effects
Chlorpromazine	12.5–25.0 mg every 2–4 h PO, PR, or IV	More sedating than haloperidol
Barbiturates Pentobarbital	60–200 mg PR every 4–8 h; loading dose of 2–3 mg/kg bolus IV, followed by 1–2 mg/kg/h continuously infused IV	Do not mix with other drugs when given IV
Phenobarbital	Loading dose of 200 mg, followed by 0.5 mg/kg/h continuously injected SQ or IV	—
Anesthetics Propofol	Begin with 2.5–5.0 μg/kg/min and titrate to desired effect every 10 min by increments of 10–20 mg/h	—

IV, intravenously; PO, per os (orally); PR, per rectum; SL, sublingually; SQ, subcutaneously.
Source: Lynch M. Palliative sedation. *Clin J Oncol Nurs.* 2003;7:653–667.

sedation. The RASS has demonstrated validity and reliability in medical and surgical, ventilated and nonventilated patients and in sedated and nonsedated adult ICU patients.[9] The RASS assessment scale is also being used in some palliative care units to assess and monitor patients undergoing mild or intermediate sedation.

Guidelines for Palliative Sedation

Institutional guidelines are important for palliative sedation so that there is a consistent standard of care and essential education for all involved practitioners. Box 4.2 is a sample checklist for palliative sedation, and Table 4.3 is a sample checklist for palliative sedation in an ICU setting.

Four factors need to be present for a patient to be considered for palliative sedation. First, the patient is terminally ill; second, the patient has severe symptoms that are refractory to treatment and intolerable to the patient, and a palliative care expert agrees that the symptoms are intractable; third, a do-not-resuscitate (DNR) order is in effect; and fourth, death is imminent (within hours to days), although this can be challenging to determine.[3] If the first three conditions exist, sedation maybe appropriate for a patient in severe distress who has been unresponsive to skilled palliative interventions. Ethics consultations or patient advocate services have been found to be useful if there is conflict about goals of care and appropriate care of someone near death, especially in the ICU setting.

Palliative Care Team

A major role of the palliative care team is to assist families in making the transition in treatment goals from cure to comfort. Refractory symptoms and the distress they cause can create a very difficult and abrupt need for this transition phase. Use of the interdisciplinary team to both plan for treatment options and participate in family meetings is critical to the success of the team. The social worker plays an important role in assessing caregiver stress and family dynamics and in coordinating family meetings. The chaplain and other psychosocial professionals provide spiritual assistance and counseling and support the decision makers through anticipatory and actual grief. The nurse is a consistent presence and skilled resource to the patient and family.

Nursing Care: Back to Basics

Communication

An important role of the nurse in the end-of-life process is to facilitate communication and establish trust between the patient, family members, and healthcare providers. Communication is vital to developing a relationship of trust and avoiding conflict during any illness, but it becomes even more important when dealing with end-of-life issues. The team must build a trusting relationship with patients and families because they make difficult decisions

Box 4.2 Palliative Sedation Checklist

Part A. Background

- Confirm patient has
  - Irreversible advanced disease
  - Apparent imminent death within hours, days, or weeks
  - A do-not-resuscitate attempt order
- Confirm that symptoms are refractory to other therapies that are acceptable to the patient and have a reasonable/practical potential to achieve comfort goals.
- Consider obtaining a peer consultation to confirm that the patient is near death with refractory symptoms.
- Complete informed consent process for palliative sedation (PS).
- Discontinue interventions not focused on comfort.
  - Discontinue routine laboratory and imaging studies.
  - Review medications, limit to those for comfort, and adjust for ease of administration (timing and route).
  - Discontinue unnecessary cardiopulmonary and vital sign monitoring.
  - Review the role of cardiac support devices (e.g., pacemaker) and disable functioning implanted defibrillators.
- Develop a plan for the use or withdrawal of nutrition and hydration during PS.
- Identify a location and an environment acceptable for providing PS.
- Use providers familiar with PS and the use of sedatives.

Part B. Treatment and Care of the Patient

- Institute and maintain aspiration precautions.
- Provide mouth care and eye protection.
- Use oxygen only for comfort, not to maintain a specific blood oxygen saturation.
- Provide medications primarily by IV or SQ route.
- Maintain bowel, bladder, and pressure point care.
- Continue, do not taper, routine opioids.
- Provide sedating medication:
  - Titrate to symptom control, not level of consciousness, using frequent reevaluation.
  - Limit vital sign monitoring to temperature and respiratory rate for dyspnea.
- Choose sedating medication based on provider experience, route available, and patient location.

Home initial dosing (choose one):

- Chlorpromazine, 25-mg suppository or 12.5-mg IV infusion every 4–6 h
- Midazolam, 0.4 mg/h by continuous IV or SQ infusion
- Lorazepam, 0.5–2.0 mg IV sublingually every 4–6 h

Hospital initial dosing (choose one):

- Chlorpromazine, 12.5–25.0 mg every 4–6 h
- Midazolam, 0.4 mg/h by continuous IV or SQ infusion
- Amobarbital or thiopental, 20 mg/h by continuous IV infusion
- Propofol, 2.5 mg/kg/min by continuous IV infusion

Source: Lynch M. Palliative sedation. *Clin J Oncol Nurs.* 2003;7:653–667.

Table 4.3 Checklist for Intensive Care Unit Personnel End-of-Life Criterion

Assessment	Met*	Not Met†
1. Determine that the primary physician, critical care physician, family, and possibly patient are in agreement with discontinuation of life-sustaining treatment.	___	___
2. Assist the family in preparation or fulfillment of familial or religious predeath rituals.	___	___
3. Place do-not-resuscitate orders on chart.	___	___
4. Provide a calm, quiet, restful atmosphere free of medical devices and technology for the patient and family, including dimming the lights in the room.	___	___
5. Turn off arrhythmia detection and turn off or decrease all auditory alarms at bedside and central station.	___	___
6. Remove all monitoring equipment from patient and patient's room except for the electrocardiograph (ECG).	___	___
7. Remove all devices unless the removal of the device would create discomfort for the patient (e.g., sequential compression device, nasogastric tube).	___	___
8. Remove or discontinue treatments that do not provide comfort to the patient.	___	___
9. Obtain orders to discontinue test and laboratory studies.	___	___
10. Liberalize visitation.	___	___
11. Notify the chaplain and social worker of end-of-life care; obtain grief packet from the chaplain.	___	___
12. Determine that family participants in the end-of-life process are present, if appropriate; place sufficient chairs in the patient's room for family members.	___	___
13. Maintain the patient's personal comfort and dignity with attention to hygiene, hairstyle, and providing moisturizers for lips and eyes.	___	___
14. Frequently assess the patient's condition, which assists in titrating medications per end-of-life protocol and level of patient discomfort.	___	___
15. Document the patient's signs and symptoms that indicate discomfort, including but not limited to the following: Agitated behavior Altered cognition Anxiety Autonomic hyperactivity Confusion Coughing Dyspnea Restlessness Self-report of symptoms Splinting Stiffness	___	___

(continued)

Table 4.3 (Continued)

Assessment	Met*	Not Met†
Tachycardia Grimacing Increased work of breathing Irritation Moaning Pain Perspiration Tachypnea Tension Trembling		
16. Remain at bedside to assess the patient for comfort or discomfort. Promptly administer sedation or analgesics. Provide emotional support to the patient and family. Ask the patient and family if additional comfort measures are needed.		
17. Obtain physician orders for additional or alterations in pain and sedation medications if the end-of-life protocol medications are ineffective in controlling the patient's discomfort.	___	___
18. Support and educate the patient's family regarding interpretation of the clinical signs and symptoms the patient may experience during the end of life.	___	___
19. Assess the family's need to be alone with the patient during and after the dying process.	___	___
20. Assess the family to determine the amount of support they require during the end-of-life process.	___	___
21. Assist the family in meeting its needs and the patient's needs for communication and final expressions of love and concern (e.g., holding a hand, talking with the patient, remembering past events).	___	___
22. Discuss signs of death and how the physician will pronounce the patient; the family will be asked to leave the room while the physician examines the patient.	___	___
23. Notify the intensive care unit physician to pronounce the patient. An ECG strip of a straight line or asystole is not needed to document the patient's death.	___	___
24. Notify the primary care physician.	___	___
25. Assist the family with decisions regarding the need for an autopsy.	___	___
26. Notify the clinical nurse specialist Monday through Friday before 3:00 p.m. to complete death paperwork.	___	___
27. Notify in-house administrator after 3:00 p.m. and on weekends to complete death paperwork.	___	___
28. Notify the chaplain, if the chaplain is not present.	___	___
29. If the patient is to have an autopsy, leave all tubes in place; if no autopsy, remove all tubes (intravenous lines may be clamped instead of removed).	___	___
30. Permit family visitation after the patient has been cleaned and tubes removed.	___	___
31. Prepare the patient for the morgue, shroud, or other.	___	___

**Met* indicates that the individual is prepared, follows suggested steps in appropriate sequence, and demonstrates minimal safe practice.

† Not met indicates that the individual is unprepared, needs repeated assistance or suggestions in order to proceed, or omits necessary steps.

Source: M. D. Anderson Cancer Center, Houston, Texas.

together. If the patient or family members do not trust the healthcare team, conflict is likely. Communication includes the following:

- Being honest and truthful
- Letting the patient and family know they will not be abandoned
- Including the patient and family in care decisions
- Helping the patient and family explore all options
- Asking the patient and family to clearly define what they need from the team
- Working to ensure that the entire team knows and understands the plan
- Practicing active listening when talking to the patient and family

In a qualitative study examining nurses' perceptions of palliative sedation, two factors made nurses more comfortable with their role in the dying process. The first was how well the nurse knew the patient as a person, and the second was the interdisciplinary team collaboration.[11]

The patient and family healthcare agent are central in the decision to use palliative sedation and need ongoing reassurance that the decision made is the right one. They may need frequent confirmation that the person is dying of the disease and that the intent of the sedation is to ensure a peaceful death but not to hasten death. The concept of "presence" with the patient and family during the death vigil is difficult to quantify but critical during periods of extreme distress. Untreated symptoms cause families and staff to be traumatized by a "horrible death." The family may fear that this "final event" will be equally traumatic. They don't want their loved one to suffer any more. They need constant explanations and reassurance about what to expect and what is happening, and the opportunity to express their grief.[8]

Physical Care

As the patient becomes more sedated, protective reflexes decrease. The ability to clear secretions decreases. This can be anticipated, and appropriate medication should be given proactively. Suctioning is kept to a minimum and only done if absolutely necessary. The blink reflex also decreases, and eyes can become dry, requiring frequent eye drops (artificial tears). Bowel and bladder management should be carefully monitored to maintain comfort. A urinary catheter is often appropriate to minimize the need for frequent changing and cleaning. Allowing the family to decide what basic comfort care they want provided to their loved one at end of life allows them some sense of control in an uncontrollable situation. Some family members may want to assist in the care of their loved one by helping with bathing, brushing the hair, and applying a lubricant to the lips; this can be quite meaningful to some family members. Other family members may prefer not to help with physical care and should be reassured that their presence alone, even if in spirit only, is equally important.

Time to Death

One of the concerns many people have with palliative sedation is that it might hasten death. Part of this concern stems from the difficulty in predicting the time of death. Several studies using different methodologies have examined effects of sedation on survival rates. The mean time to death in a large four-country study ranged from 1.9 to 3.2 days,[5] and the median time to death in a Taiwanese study was 5 days.[12] A study of patients in Japanese hospices indicated that sedating medications did not shorten life span.[13] However, because of ethical considerations, none of these studies was a controlled trial, so it is not possible to determine whether sedation may or may not result in hastening the death. In situations of unbearable distress, sedation remains an appropriate option to relieve suffering.

Ethical Considerations Concerning Palliative Sedation

Palliative sedation is a medical therapy for the imminently dying when pain and suffering are intolerable and other interventions have proved inadequate. Intent is the critical issue and separates palliative sedation at end of life from assisted dying and euthanasia. With sedation, the intent is to produce somnolence and relieve suffering, not hasten death. In assisted dying—where the intent is to produce death to relieve suffering—the agent is the patient. In euthanasia—where the intent is to produce death to relieve suffering—the agent is another person. The ethical and legal principles that apply to palliative sedation are patient autonomy (patient's choice), beneficence (do good), nonmaleficence (do no harm), and the principle of double effect.

In 1997, the U.S. Supreme Court ruled unanimously that "there is no constitutional right to physician-assisted suicide" but "terminal sedation is intended for symptom relief and not assisted suicide . . . and is appropriate in the aggressive practice of palliative care."[14] The Hospice and Palliative Nurses Association has issued a Position Paper in support of palliative sedation.[15] The use of palliative sedation for existential suffering remains controversial.

Informed Consent

Informed consent is always a process. A patient's symptoms may have been difficult to control over time and may have escalated as the patient's disease has progressed. Patients (or their agents when they cannot speak for themselves) must always be involved in these decisions. Palliative sedation involves an important trade-off between symptom control and alertness, and different patients will weigh this differently. The need for sedation may be a palliative care emergency to relieve distress, in which case consent would be similar to obtaining consent in any other emergency situation. A family meeting to discuss the situation would then follow.

A family meeting includes a well-planned, compassionate, and clear discussion with the patient and family about the patient's goals and values in the setting of end-of-life care. The bedside nurse is an important participant in these meetings to provide insight into the care and support needed by the family. It is important to plan these meetings carefully if at all possible to ensure that the appropriate family members are present. Allowing the designated decision maker to invite significant people to the planned meeting allows key participants to hear the information at the same time. A religious or spiritual representative can be helpful at these meetings, if the family so desires.

The primary physician usually begins the family meeting with a brief, clear report on the current condition of the patient. Supporting documentation of the current condition, such as recent laboratory data or other diagnostic test results, may be helpful to some families. The patient and family should be provided all the time necessary to raise concerns, clarify information, and have their questions answered. The same questions may be raised time and time again to different team members, and they need to be answered with consistent information to reduce uncertainty. Next, the treatment options should be discussed. When discussing terminal sedation options, it is important to assess the patient's and family's cultural and religious beliefs and concerns.

Documentation in the chart should include the parties present, the reason for sedation (symptom distress), and the primary goal (patient comfort), as well as patient terminal status, notation of any professional consultations, documentation that the patient is near death and has refractory symptoms, planned discontinuance of treatments not focused on comfort, plan regarding hydration and nutrition, and anticipated risks or burdens of sedation.[8] Either at the end of the family meeting or the next day in nonemergency cases, some institutions require that an informed consent document is signed by the patient, family, or healthcare agent. Because it usually is not possible to communicate verbally with the sedated patient, it is important to make sure that the patient and family are given time to talk with each other and say goodbye, if that is possible, before proceeding with sedation. A well-planned family meeting decreases miscommunication and supports the family during a difficult decision-making time by allowing all pertinent parties to hear the same information at the same time. The decision for palliative sedation is made by the patient, family, and healthcare agent with guidance from the palliative care team.

The Nurse Caregiver

In a literature review examining the experience of nurses caring for terminally ill patients in ICU settings, several barriers related to provision of terminal care were identified: (1) lack of involvement in the plan of care and comfort; (2) disagreement among physicians and other healthcare team members; (3) inadequacy of pain relief; (4) unrealistic expectations of families; (5) personal difficulty coping; (6) lack of experience and education; (7) staffing levels; and (8) environmental circumstances.[16] In a Japanese study of 2,607 nurses involved in palliative sedation, 37% reported that they wanted to leave their current jobs because of the burden of palliative sedation; 12% reported that their involvement in palliative sedation made them feel helpless; and 11% would avoid a patient who is being treated with palliative sedation if possible. This study concluded that a significant number of nurses feel serious emotional burdens related to palliative sedation.[17]

Nurses who work with patients requiring palliative sedation are at increased risk for burnout if not intimately involved with the team decision-making process.

In addition, if left out of decision-making processes such as the team planning and family conferences, they are denied the information needed for effective counseling at the patient's bedside. Formal and informal support systems for nurses, as well as education in end-of-life care, spiritual support, and individual support, are essential.

An interdisciplinary team meeting after the death of the patient can function as both a learning experience and a debriefing session. Working in an environment that recognizes the need for support and education of staff, as well as the importance of mentors and advance practice nurses, allows nurses to face these challenges as they arise.

Conclusion

Although nurses and other healthcare practitioners may disagree about what is a "good death," there is general agreement about what is a "bad death." Palliative sedation is a necessary option for a small number of patients with refractory and intolerable symptoms and suffering at end of life. These options are part of the spectrum of palliative care and are ethically and legally supported. However, the ability to determine refractoriness of symptoms can be complicated and is largely dependent on the skills of the practitioner and the tools available to manage complex symptoms. Nurses have a central role in ensuring that a dying patient undergoing palliative sedation has his or her symptoms well controlled and that the family members are well supported. Education of palliative care nurses in these areas is essential.

References

1. Hall MJ, Levant S, DeFrances CJ. Trends in inpatient hospital deaths: National Hospital Discharge Survey, 2000–2010. NCHS data brief, no 118. Hyattsville, MD: National Center for Health Statistics; 2013.
2. Aungst H. "Death with dignity." The first decade of Oregon's physician-assisted death act. *Geriatrics*. 2008;63:20–24.
3. Lynch M. Palliative sedation. *Clin J Oncol Nurs*. 2003;7:653–667.
4. Claessens P, Menten J, Schotsmans P, Broeckaert B. Palliative sedation: a review of the research literature. *J Pain Symptom Manage*. 2008;36(3):310–333.
5. Fainsinger RL, Waller A, Bercovici M, et al. A multicentre international study of sedation for uncontrolled symptoms in terminally ill patients. *Palliat Med*. 2000;14:257–265.
6. Cherney N. Sedation for the care of patients with advanced cancer. *Nat Clin Pract Oncol*. 2006;3(9):492–500.
7. Ganzini L, Dobscha SK, Heintz RT, Press N. Oregon physicians' perceptions of patients who request assisted suicide and their families. *J Palliat Med*. 2003;6:381–390.
8. Cowan JD, Palmer TW. Practical guide to palliative sedation. *Curr Oncol Rep*. 2002;4:242–249.

9. Sessler CN, Jo Grap M, Ramsay MA. Evaluating and monitoring analgesia and sedation in the intensive care unit. *Crit Care*. 2008;12(Suppl 3):15.
10. Troug RD, Campbell M, Curtis JR, et al. Recommendations for end-of-life care in the intensive care unit: a consensus statement by the American College of Critical Care Medicine. *Crit Care Med*. 2008;36:953–963.
11. Beel AC, Hawranik PG, McClement S, Daeninck P. Palliative sedation: nurses' perceptions. *Int J Palliat Nurs*. 2006;12(11):510–518.
12. Chiu TY, Hu WY, Lue BH, et al. Sedation for refractory symptoms of terminal cancer patients in Taiwan. *J Pain Symptom Manage*. 2001;21:467–472.
13. Morita T, Tsunoda J, Inoue S, Chihara S. Effects of high-dose opioids and sedatives on survival in terminally ill cancer patients. *J Pain Symptom Manage*. 2001;21:282–289.
14. Burt RA. The Supreme Court speaks: not assisted suicide but a constitutional right to palliative care. *N Engl J Med*. 1997;337:1234–1236.
15. Hospice and Palliative Nurses Association. Position paper: Palliative sedation at the end of life.2011. http://hpna.advancingexpertcare.org/wp-content/uploads/2014/09/Palliative-Sedation-PositionStatement-080311.pdf. Accessed July 7, 2015.
16. Espinosa L, Young E, Walsh T. Barriers to ICU nurses providing terminal care: an integrated literature review. *Crit Care Nurse*. 2008;31:83–93.
17. Morita T, Miyashita M, Kimura R, et al. Emotional burden of nurses in palliative sedation therapy. *Palliat Med*. 2004;18:550–557.

Chapter 5

Withdrawal of Life-Sustaining Therapies

Mechanical Ventilation, Dialysis, and Cardiac Devices

Margaret L. Campbell and Linda M. Gorman

Benefits and Burdens of Mechanical Ventilation

Mechanical ventilation (MV) has been used for decades to support breathing when patients experienced acute or chronic respiratory failure. MV is of benefit when the patient, for a number of reasons, cannot maintain normal ventilation, as evidenced by increasing carbon dioxide and respiratory acidosis, and invasive and noninvasive modalities are then employed. Invasive MV is accomplished after the establishment of an artificial airway such as an endotracheal tube or tracheostomy. Noninvasive MV is applied over the nose or nose and mouth through a tight-fitting facemask.

Invasive MV is employed after cardiopulmonary arrest, during general anesthesia, to treat respiratory failure that is not responsive to noninvasive ventilation, and in patients who are ventilator dependent. Endotracheal intubation is used for periods of less than 2 weeks of ventilation; continued ventilation after 2 weeks is supported by tracheostomy. When respiratory failure occurs during an exacerbation of chronic pulmonary disease, noninvasive ventilation is often useful as a first response.[1] Patients with obstructive sleep apnea, chronic obstructive pulmonary disease, and amyotrophic lateral sclerosis often use noninvasive ventilation at night or when breathing is difficult during the day.

Patients often experience discomfort during MV. With noninvasive modalities, the tight-fitting mask may produce generalized pressure-associated discomfort, feelings of suffocation, and pressure lesions on the bridge of the nose. Endotracheal intubation causes gagging, coughing, and drooling and leaves the patient unable to speak because the tube passes through the vocal cords. In many cases of endotracheal intubation and some cases of noninvasive ventilation, the patient requires mechanical restraints or sedation to maintain the integrity of the life-saving treatment and to ensure ventilator synchrony.

Ventilator-dependent patients experience fewer burdens because they are routinely ventilated through a tracheostomy. Nonetheless, chronic ventilator dependence limits patient mobility and contributes to the development of immobility complications such as pressure ulcers, deep vein thrombosis, and pneumonia.

Ventilator withdrawal is considered a treatment option when the treatment is more burdensome than beneficial, such as when the patient has a terminal illness or is unconscious or when the patient makes an informed, capable decision to cease treatment because his or her quality of life is poor.[2] In critical care units (adult, pediatric, and neonatal), ventilator withdrawal is usually undertaken because the patient is not expected to survive or to regain functional consciousness. Clinical standards, policies, and procedures about foregoing life-sustaining therapy, including MV, are in wide use and reflect broad agreement about the underlying principles regarding these decisions.

Although withdrawal of ventilation occurs on a frequent basis across settings of care, there is little empirical evidence to guide the process. A review of the evidence to guide a ventilator withdrawal process demonstrated that small samples and largely retrospective chart reviews characterize the body of evidence about processes for ventilator withdrawal.[2] The cited research is not adequately conclusive to make recommendations in all cases of ventilator withdrawal. However, a number of suggested processes may be useful in this clinical context, along with a team approach to the procedure and patient care to address anticipated symptoms.

Patients are ventilated because of respiratory failure and an inability to exchange respiratory gases without mechanical support. Dyspnea arises from increased inspiratory effort, hypercarbia, or hypoxemia; dyspnea is anticipated during and after ventilator withdrawal. Prevention and alleviation of dyspnea or respiratory distress becomes the focus of care during ventilator withdrawal. Some patients, if awake, may experience fear or anxiety before or during ventilator withdrawal, which will require attention if present. Adult patients may experience barotrauma to the trachea from the pressure in the cuff, leading to laryngeal edema or spasm after extubation with development of post-extubation stridor.

Ventilator Withdrawal Processes

Advance Preparation

The Centers for Medicare and Medicaid Services has enacted guidelines for consistent processes around organ donation.[3] Hospital staff must notify their state organ procurement organization (OPO) when decisions about ventilator withdrawal are being considered. The OPO will collaborate with the hospital staff to identify whether the patient is a candidate for donation after cardiac death and to seek consent from the next of kin. This evaluation by the OPO must be completed before ventilation is withdrawn.

Timing to conduct the withdrawal process is generally negotiated with the patient's family and the healthcare team. This timing depends on which team members will be present, including support personnel such as a chaplain. The time needs to be communicated to all clinical team members, and ideally the assigned nurse should have a reduced assignment to be able to spend time with the patient and family.

Not all family members want to be present at the bedside during withdrawal. Another room nearby can be arranged with adequate seating, tissues, water, and access to a telephone. Religious observances or family-specific rituals need to be accommodated and completed before beginning the withdrawal process. Patient and family questions about what to expect can be addressed before beginning the process. When ventilation is withdrawn from a small child, infant, or neonate, it is customary for a parent to hold the child on his or her lap during the process.

Neuromuscular blocking agents (NMBAs) are being used with less frequency in the intensive care unit (ICU), but when they are used, it is impossible to assess the patient's comfort. Thus, the NMBA should be discontinued with evidence of patient neuromuscular recovery before ventilator withdrawal is undertaken. In some cases, the duration of action of these agents is prolonged, such as when the patient has liver or renal failure and impaired clearance. Therefore, although controversial, withdrawal can proceed with careful attention to ensuring patient comfort if an unacceptable delay in withdrawing MV occurs because of protracted effects of an NMBA.

Measuring Distress

Dyspnea, also known as breathlessness, is a nociceptive phenomenon defined as "a subjective experience of breathing discomfort that consists of qualitatively distinct sensations that vary in intensity. The experience derives from interactions among multiple physiological, psychological, social and environmental factors, and may induce secondary physiological and behavioral responses."[4] Dyspnea can be perceived and verified only by the person experiencing it. Many patients who are undergoing ventilator withdrawal are cognitively impaired or unconscious as a result of underlying neurologic lesions or hemodynamic, metabolic, or respiratory dysfunction that produces cognitive impairment or unconsciousness. Respiratory distress is an observable (behavioral) corollary to dyspnea; the physical and emotional suffering that results from the experience of asphyxiation is characterized by behaviors that can be observed and measured.

Most patients undergoing ventilator withdrawal will be unable to provide a self-report about any dyspnea experienced, particularly patients who are unconscious or severely cognitively impaired, infants, and neonates. Attempts to elicit a self-report should be made if the patient is conscious. Skill is required to detect nuances of behaviors, particularly when the patient is unable to validate the nurse's assessment. Initiation and escalation of sedatives and opioids should be guided by patient behaviors.

The Respiratory Distress Observation Scale is suitable for assessing the adult patient during the withdrawal of mechanical ventilation; reliability and validity have been established.[5] This eight-variable categorical scale is the only known tool for assessing respiratory distress when the patient cannot self-report dyspnea, as typifies most patients undergoing ventilator withdrawal. Infants and neonates often display nasal flaring, grunting at end-expiration, and sternal retraction. Brain-dead patients by definition will not show distress, cough, gag, or breathe during or after ventilator withdrawal, and sedation or analgesia is not indicated.

Premedication for Anticipated Distress

As is the standard with pain management, opioids should be initiated to signs of distress, and the advice to "start low and titrate slowly" is sage. For the opioid-naïve adult, an initial bolus of 3 to 5 mg of morphine is recommended. Pediatric dosing is usually initiated at 0.1 to 0.2 mg/kg.[6] Anticipatory premedication is a sound practice if distress is already evident or can be anticipated. There is no justification for medicating a brain-dead patient, and one could argue that the patient in coma with only minimal brainstem function is also unlikely to experience distress. Doses that correspond to customary dosing for the treatment of dyspnea should guide dosing during ventilator withdrawal. Documentation of the signs of distress and rationale for dose escalation is important to ensure continuity across professional caregivers and to prevent overmedication and the appearance of hastening death. At the conclusion of the process, a continuous infusion may be initiated to maintain patient comfort; an infusion rate equivalent to 50% of the total amount of bolus medication is recommended. Thus, if the patient received three boluses at 5 mg (15 mg), the infusion would start at a rate of 7.5 mg/hour.

Weaning Method

Terminal extubation is characterized by ceasing ventilatory support and removing the endotracheal tube in one step. Terminal weaning is a process of stepwise, gradual reductions in oxygen and ventilation, terminating with placement on a T-piece or with extubation. There are no known investigations comparing one method to another.[2]

With no comparative evidence to support one method over another, it is difficult to make a recommendation. Rapid terminal weaning may afford the clinician the most control because it allows for careful, sequential adjustments to the ventilator, with precise titration of medications to ensure patient comfort. Continuous patient monitoring with readily accessible opioids and sedatives will afford the patient and family comfort regardless of method employed.

Extubation Considerations

Patients who are ventilator dependent are generally ventilated through a tracheostomy tube. After ventilator withdrawal, a tracheostomy mask with humidified room air or low-flow oxygen can be placed. Patients experiencing acute respiratory failure are ventilated through a nasal or oral endotracheal tube. Adult tubes have a cuff to maintain tube placement and occlude the trachea to prevent air leaking and loss of tidal volume; neonatal tubes are cuffless.

Removal of the endotracheal tube should be performed whenever possible because of patient comfort and the aesthetic appearance of the patient. However, in some cases airway compromise can be anticipated, such as when the patient has a swollen, protuberant tongue or has no gag or cough reflexes. In cases of airway compromise, the disconcerting noises may be more distressing to the attendant family than the presence of the tube. Medication with dexamethasone may reduce airway edema, permitting extubation when patients are at high risk for post-extubation laryngeal edema, but dosing would need to start 12 hours before withdrawal if the timing permits. A cuff-leak test entails measuring the volume of air loss when the endotracheal tube cuff is deflated before extubation. Air loss of less than 140 cc predicts post-extubation stridor. Aerosolized racemic epinephrine is a useful intervention to reduce stridor after extubation. Family counseling about usual noises that can be expected and that should cause no distress is done before extubation.

Oxygen

A growing body of evidence suggests that oxygen is a useful palliative intervention to treat dyspnea when the patient is experiencing distress and is hypoxemic but has no benefit when the patient has normal oxygenation. Further, when patients are near death and in no distress, oxygen is not necessary. Thus, the patient can be cared for without oxygen following ventilator withdrawal unless there are signs of respiratory distress and hypoxemia. Nasal cannula is better tolerated than a facemask if oxygen is initiated.

Dialysis Discontinuation

Benefits and Burdens of Dialysis

Dialysis was introduced as a treatment for end-stage renal disease (ESRD) in 1962. In the early years, the number of patients receiving dialysis was limited by the small number of dialysis machines available, and only individuals younger than 40 years of age, family breadwinners, and those without severe medical problems like diabetes were considered. In 1973, Medicare established universal entitlement for chronic dialysis; currently more than 300,000 Americans receive dialysis.[7] ESRD, which is also referred to as *chronic kidney disease* (CKD) stage 5, is defined as a glomerular filtration rate of less than 15 mL/minute (normal, ≥90 mL/minute). The most common causes include diabetes mellitus, heart failure, hypertension, and glomerulonephritis. Acute renal failure, also known as *acute kidney injury* (AKI), is commonly seen in critically ill patients who suffer from dehydration, sepsis, hypotension, or trauma; AKI may lead to dialysis.

In the past 10 years, the dialysis population has changed. The current dialysis population is older with more comorbidities, higher symptom burden, and a higher mortality rate than previous populations. More than 75% of hemodialysis patients are older than 65 years. Patients older than 80 years now constitute the fastest growing segment of this population and have a 46% mortality rate in the first year of dialysis. The cause of this change in population is multifactorial and may be advances in life-prolonging therapies, nephrologists' focus on "life-saving" approaches, and reports that nephrologists are increasingly being expected to dialyze patients whom they believe may receive little benefit from this therapy.[8] This population will not be candidates for transplantation, so they will remain on dialysis until they die or until it is discontinued. As expected, elderly patients tend to have high symptom burden, higher rates of rehospitalization within 30 days of discharge, and frequent ICU admissions, as well as higher use of more intensive procedures than younger patients.[7] They also may have slower progression of renal disease, which should also be taken into consideration before rushing to start dialysis.

A decision to stop dialysis is a frequent occurrence, especially in a frail elderly population. The nephrology community has been moving to address improved quality of life and incorporating advances from the palliative care field. Renal and palliative care experts recommend incorporating a discussion about discontinuing dialysis in the informed consent process for dialysis routinely with this population and revisiting it regularly as the patient declines. National initiatives, including the Renal Physicians Association Clinical Practice Guidelines, are addressing the growing needs of this older, sicker population[9] (Box 5.1). Using well-established ethical principles and processes, the ethical framework of shared decision making as covered in these guidelines gives support to the nephrologist to address the appropriate use of dialysis.

Symptoms of uremia are usually controlled quickly with dialysis; paradoxically, dialysis produces one of the highest symptom burden as well as hospitalization rates of any chronic illness population. Jablonski found an average of six uncomfortable symptoms while on dialysis.[10] Davison and Jhangri found a mean of seven symptoms, and more than 50% of patients had chronic pain.[11] Other discomforts with dialysis include fatigue, pruritus, constipation, anorexia, anxiety, and sleep disturbances. Frail elderly patients with multiple comorbidities receiving dialysis are particularly vulnerable to a high symptom burden. Therefore, although life may be prolonged with dialytic management of uremia, this population's quality of life will often not improve. Thus, a trial of dialysis may be offered in some cases to elderly patients to see whether dialysis will improve symptoms, although this will require vascular access. Germain and colleagues have noted that a time-limited trial of dialysis is appropriate only if there is a reasonable chance it will provide a net benefit to the patient and achieve the patient's and family's goals.[8] Some investigators are finding that patients have poor self-reported knowledge of options in stage 5 CKD and that many regretted their decision to start dialysis. Others have found that dialysis patients tended to be more optimistic about prognosis than their nephrologists, indicating that these patients had not been given accurate information or had not absorbed this information.

In response to the aging population and trends of dialyzing older and sicker patients, interest is growing in nondialytic alternatives for ESRD. Conservative management of uremia without dialysis is now being offered more frequently in the presence of advanced age and comorbidities.[8] Conservative treatment is associated with a high symptom burden, so concomitant palliative care is indicated.[12]

Box 5.1 Renal Physicians Association Guidelines on Initiation and Withdrawal From Dialysis[9]

1. Develop a physician-patient relationship for shared decision making.
2. Fully inform acute kidney disease (AKI), stage 4 and 5 chronic kidney disease (CKD), and end-stage renal disease (ESRD) patients about their dialysis, prognosis, and all treatment options.
3. Give all patients with AKI, stage 5 CKD, or ESRD an estimate of prognosis specific to their overall condition.
4. Institute advance care planning.
5. If appropriate, forgo (withhold initiating or withdraw ongoing) dialysis for patients with AKI, CKD, or ESRD in certain well-defined situations.
6. Consider forgoing dialysis for AKI, CKD, or ESRD patients who have a very poor prognosis or for whom dialysis cannot be provided safely, as in advanced dementia or unstable hypotension.
7. Consider a time-limited trial of dialysis for patients who require dialysis but have an uncertain prognosis, or for whom a consensus cannot be reached about providing dialysis.
8. Establish a systematic, due-process approach to conflict resolution if there is disagreement about what decision should be made with regard to dialysis.
9. To improve patient-centered outcomes, offer palliative care services and interventions to all AKI, CKD, and ESRD patients who suffer from burdens of their disease.
10. Use a systematic approach to communicate about diagnosis, prognosis, treatment options, and goals of care.

Source: Renal Physicians Association. *Shared Decision-Making in the Appropriate Initiation of and Withdrawal From Dialysis: Clinical Practice Guidelines.* 2nd ed. Rockville, MD; Renal Physicians Association; 2010.

Discontinuing Dialysis

Dialysis was rarely withdrawn in the early years unless there was loss of vascular access that made dialysis impossible. Today, 20% to 25% of patients receiving dialysis have it discontinued each year.[9] Stopping dialysis remains the second leading condition before death in this population.[7] Stopping dialysis should be considered when the burdens of dialysis outweigh the benefits, dialysis is no longer serving to substantially prolong life, or it is only prolonging death.

The most common reason for stopping dialysis is unacceptable quality of life. Specific causes include pain, burden of multiple symptoms, acute complications such as infection, technical problems with dialysis, dementia, stroke, and cancer. Additionally, some patients become too unstable to complete the dialysis session. Peritoneal dialysis patients may be too sick to carry out exchanges and need to obtain vascular access for hemodialysis. Inserting new access lines may cause the patient to reconsider discontinuing dialysis.

Addressing symptom burden, including psychological symptoms, is an important consideration before making the decision to discontinue dialysis. Patients on dialysis often struggle with depression, changes in body image, sexual dysfunction, loss of control, irritability, and dependency issues along with the physical symptoms. These can all contribute to a patient's consideration of stopping dialysis. When discontinuation is being considered, addressing symptom burden is key before stopping dialysis.[13] A thorough assessment and interventions to address all these issues should be part of any treatment plan when discontinuing dialysis is being considered. See Box 5.2 for guidelines on this decision. A discussion that includes the patient, family, and nephrologist about the burdens, benefits, possible reversible factors, goals, and outcomes needs to be part of the treatment plan when considering the option of discontinuing dialysis. If the patient cannot make his or her own decisions, surrogate decision makers must be driven by the patient's values.

When patients make their own decisions, stopping dialysis can be a freeing, almost euphoric experience. The patient usually has a few days before uremic symptoms begin, and this time can include eating favorite, formerly forbidden foods and opportunities to say goodbye to loved ones. This allows a patient to maintain some sense of control over his or her life and the dying process. Choosing the date of the last dialysis, where to spend the last days, and what foods to eat can enhance a sense of control. Family members may struggle with accepting the patient's choice. Loved ones need to be prepared that the patient may become cognitively impaired suddenly as the creatinine rises.

Box 5.2 Guidelines for Making Dialysis Discontinuation Decisions

- Identify patients who may benefit from discontinuation, including those patients with poor prognosis, poor quality of life, pain that is poorly responsive to treatment, progressive untreatable disease, and technically difficult dialysis.
  - Address patient's decision-making capacity.
- Discuss goals with patient and family.
- Discuss quality of life.
- Discuss possible symptoms and their palliation.
  - Identify possible reversible causes.
- Clarify that dialysis discontinuation is an option, as part of review of treatment modalities, when educating patients who are new to dialysis.
- Provide reassurance of a peaceful death.
- Allow time for discussion.
- Make the recommendation to stop dialysis and request family assent.

Source: Davison SN, Rosielle DA. Withdrawal of dialysis: decision making #207. *J Palliat Med.* 2012;15:1270–1271.

When the patient is unable to participate in decision making because of dementia, delirium, or critical illness, families and surrogates often struggle with making this literally life-and-death decision. But if the patient's suffering with dialysis has been evident, it can be easier to make the decision to stop. Another key factor for surrogates is the patient's inability to return to an acceptable quality of life.

Treating Symptoms After Discontinuation

Death after discontinuation of dialysis generally occurs in 8 to 12 days, although patients with many comorbidities may die sooner, and patients who make urine will live longer. Nearly all patients discontinuing dialysis die within 1 month. Death is generally caused by accumulation of toxins, including potassium, as well as other factors due to comorbidities. Patients may have a few days of relative comfort with sudden onset of symptoms. Last days and hours are characterized by hypersomnolence followed by coma. A peaceful death can be achieved with palliative care management of symptoms. Cohen and colleagues found that most families whose loved one died after withdrawal of dialysis rated the death as good to very good.[14]

The most frequent symptoms after discontinuation include pain, delirium, dyspnea, nausea, and itching. Frequent pain assessment and aggressive analgesia are important because symptoms can develop quickly. Although uremia itself is painless, patients may experience pain from their general medical condition. Morphine should be avoided because of its metabolite morphine-3-glucuronide, which increases with kidney failure, putting the patient at risk for myoclonus, seizures, and hyperalgesia. Fentanyl and methadone are better choices. Hydromorphone and oxycodone can be used but with caution. Hydromorphone does have a metabolite that can accumulate, and oxycodone has not been well studied in this population.[8] Myoclonus can be treated with benzodiazepines if it occurs. As the patient becomes obtunded near death, swallowing a pill may become difficult, and liquid opioids may be selected. Methadone can be given as an elixir into the sublingual or buccal space, where it will gradually trickle into the pharynx and be swallowed.

Delirium, confusion, and somnolence are expected as part of the uremic syndrome. A more severe form of delirium called *uremic encephalopathy* occurs infrequently. It is characterized by extreme agitation and hallucinations. Haloperidol, clonazepam, or lorazepam is useful if the patient becomes agitated, and the dose is not dependent on renal function.

Dyspnea can occur from fluid retention and pleural effusion. Anticholinergics to reduce oral secretions, opioids for dyspnea, and low-flow oxygen may be helpful. Stopping artificial hydration and nutrition will minimize fluid retention. Pulmonary edema is a palliative care emergency that may arise from volume overload. Diuresis is not possible, but systemic vasodilation may provide relief; nitroglycerin paste every 6 hours is recommended. Ultrafiltration through the dialysis access, if patent and if the patient is still in the hospital, will also relieve volume overload.

Nausea may be an effect of uremia, and delayed gastric emptying is common in ESRD; haloperidol is a useful antiemetic in this context. The liberty to

Box 5.3 Treatment Principles When Discontinuing Dialysis

- Avoid volume overload, including hydration and artificial nutrition.
- Use symptom management medications not metabolized by the kidneys.
- Discontinue all non-symptom-management medications to reduce risk for toxicities.
- Involve a pharmacist consultation early to ensure that no medications given are metabolized by the kidneys.
- Anticipate common symptoms and have appropriate medications available because symptoms can occur suddenly.
- Prepare patient and family for what to expect, especially addressing common unfounded fears of drowning in fluid.

eat previously forbidden foods may contribute to the onset of nausea and vomiting, and the patient will need to be counseled about moderation.

Itching, referred to as *uremic pruritus*, is another effect of uremia and responds well to benzodiazepines and diphenhydramine, along with lanolin-based or capsaicin creams. Principles for treating uremic symptoms are provided in Box 5.3. Symptom management strategies need to be in place when dialysis is stopped because the time frame to death is brief and symptoms can intensify quickly.

Role of Palliative Care and Hospice

Dialysis centers are encouraged to develop a palliative care approach to address their patients' needs, which may include advance care planning for timing of discontinuation of dialysis and location of death. Germain, Davison, and Moss,[8] leaders in nephrology, recommend that palliative care should be offered to all patients with ESRD who experience burdens of their disease regardless of whether they start or refuse dialysis therapy and whether they continue or withdraw from dialysis therapy. Palliative care consultation is especially important with complex pain and symptom management.

Hospice care can also be appropriate both for dialysis patients with comorbidities and patients who are considering discontinuing dialysis; however, hospice has historically been underutilized in this population. The percentage of dying ESRD patients who receive hospice is significantly less than patients with other diagnoses. (See Box 5.4 for a list of barriers to hospice utilization.) Hospice care is appropriate for patients when dialysis is stopped. Making a referral to hospice early in the discussion period about stopping dialysis may increase access earlier. Hospice can help these patients remain at home after dialysis is stopped and manage symptoms effectively. Patients may also qualify for hospice while continuing on dialysis because of their poor prognosis and comorbidities in some cases when they have a second terminal diagnosis in addition to ESRD, such as heart failure.[8] These patients can benefit from improved symptom management and ongoing discussion about goals.

Box 5.4 Barriers to Use of Hospice in Patients With End-Stage Renal Disease

Financial disincentives and confusion about coverage and eligibility

Hospice agencies and local dialysis centers that often do not have relationships

Hospice agencies' concern about reimbursement when the patient is still on dialysis

Nephrology professionals not addressing end-of-life issues with patients

Dialysis staff often with inaccurate information about hospice care

Patients and families with lack of awareness of life-limiting nature of end-stage renal disease

Hospice not offered when dialysis is being discontinued because of brief life expectancy

Nephrologists who are often driven by "life-saving" culture

Lack of good prognostic models for patients remaining on dialysis who also qualify for hospice

Sources: Germain MJ, Davison SN, Moss AH. When enough is enough: the nephrologist's responsibility in ordering dialysis treatments. *Am J Kidney Dis.* 2011;58:135–143.

Deactivation of Cardiac Implantable Devices

Benefits and Burdens of Cardiac Assist Devices

Implantable cardioverter-defibrillators (ICDs), pacemakers, ventricular assist devices (VADs), and even a totally artificial replacement heart used for many patients with advanced cardiac disease represent advanced life-sustaining technology. The number of adult patients with implantable cardiac devices is rising sharply, making it among the most common cardiovascular devices used in contemporary clinical practice.[15] Because these devices reduce the incidence of sudden death, patients with implantable defibrillators are more likely to die from other nonarrhythmic causes, such as cancer, lung disease, advanced dementia, and congestive heart failure.

Discussions About Deactivation of Devices

Before insertion of an ICD, pacemaker, or VAD, a general discussion should occur with the patient and family regarding the possibility that the device may be deactivated at a future point in time if therapy is ineffective, no longer needed, or not desired. During the informed consent process, information is provided to the patient about the device, its indications, how it works, the expected benefits, the risks, required follow-up, device maintenance (e.g., battery changes), and the possibility that the device may be deactivated in the future. A statement such as the following introduces the topic: "A time may come in the future when the device may not work as we had anticipated, or you may decide that you no longer want it. If that time comes we will talk about deactivating the device." When having end-of-life "discussions with patients and their families facing the last chapter, it is easier if they have heard previously of the potential circumstances for turning the defibrillation off."

Grassman reported, "We had a patient who went home with hospice care. The ICD was never turned off. As a result, the wife told us that the patient died in her arms while the defibrillator jolted him 33 times before the battery ran down."[16] Thus, not addressing deactivation of the ICD can cause not only unnecessary suffering for the patient but also distress for the patient's family. Even when death is expected and discussions have occurred regarding resuscitation and other end-of-life care, the topic of deactivating the ICD is not routinely discussed.

Deactivation Procedures

Pacemakers

A pacemaker is intended to correct an abnormal heart rate or rhythm. Some patients are only mildly reliant on the device; others are total dependent to the extent that if the pacemaker is deactivated, discomfort secondary to complete heart block or bradycardia can occur. Sudden death at the time of disabling the pacemaker is unlikely, unless the patient is pacemaker dependent.

Trained personnel should interrogate the pacemaker with the pacemaker programmer. The clinician should prepare the patient and family for a rapid death after deactivation if the patient is pacemaker dependent. The pacemaker settings (e.g., rate and output) are adjusted so that pacing does not occur—this can be done gradually or all at once. The patient can be premedicated with an anxiolytic or sedative if desired, particularly if a relatively sudden death can be anticipated and the patient is capable of experiencing distress.

Implantable Cardioverter-Defibrillators

Defibrillators are intended only to convert a lethal ventricular arrhythmia. Deactivation of an ICD will not degrade quality of life or create discomfort. Conversely, as illustrated previously, ICD firing while the patient is dying can be distressing to both the patient and family.

Deactivation should be done by trained personnel using the programmer for either device. A pacemaker magnet can be placed over the ICD generator, palpable under the skin, to deactivate when an ICD programmer is unavailable. However, it will not deactivate the backup pacing function of the ICD; this can only be done by an ICD programmer. The funeral director will need to be informed about the presence of the device or any other implanted metallic device, especially one with a battery, if cremation is planned.

Ventricular Assist Devices

VADs are mechanical pumps surgically implanted to improve the performance of the damaged left (LVAD), right (RVAD), or both (BiVAD) ventricles. VADs can be used short-term as a bridge to recovery or transplantation or as destination therapy, that is, as an alternative to transplantation. Short-term support is indicated for patients who develop cardiogenic shock in which recovery is anticipated with devices outside the body attached to large consoles. The average duration of VAD support for these critically ill patients is 1 week, but the units are capable of providing support for up to 1 month. Prolonged support is associated with coagulopathy, thrombocytopenia, thromboembolism, and hemolysis. When VADs are inserted as destination therapy, it is expected that the patient will need the VAD for the rest of his or her life, so the VAD is considered a final treatment. Technologic advances have made VADs compact and portable, allowing freedom for patients to be discharged home from the hospital with high-level home health follow-up. Initial clinical trials of older pulsatile-flow VADs showed a 52% 1-year survival rate; more recent studies of continuous flow pumps demonstrated a 73% 1-year survival rate.[17] Trained personnel should stop the VAD after patient and family preparation and silencing of the device alarms. The patient may experience distress from heart failure and may benefit from premedication with a diuretic and an anxiolytic. After deactivation, the patient will require close monitoring and symptomatic treatment of heart failure until death occurs.

Summary

Withdrawal of mechanical ventilation, discontinuation of dialysis, and deactivation of cardiac devices are procedures that occur with relative frequency. The benefits of these therapies are to replace failing organs, extend life, and improve quality of life by relieving symptom distress associated with organ failure. When the burdens exceed the benefits, or when the patient is near death or unresponsive, decisions may be made to cease these therapies.

In some cases, such as ICD deactivation, no distress is anticipated. In others, such as discontinuing dialysis or withdrawing MV, measures to palliate anticipated distress must be applied. A peaceful death after cessation of life-prolonging therapies can be provided.

References

1. Azoulay E, Kouatchet A, Jaber S, et al. Noninvasive mechanical ventilation in patients having declined tracheal intubation. *Intensive Care Med.* 2013;39:292–301.
2. Campbell ML. How to withdraw mechanical ventilation: a systematic review of the literature. *AACN Adv Crit Care*. 2007;18:397-403; quiz 344–345.
3. Hospital conditions of participation about organ/tissue donation. http://www.cms.gov/manuals/downloads/som107ap_a_hospitals.pdf. Accessed July 7, 2015.
4. Parshall MB, Schwartzstein RM, Adams L, et al. An official American Thoracic Society statement: update on the mechanisms, assessment, and management of dyspnea. *Am J Respir Crit Care Med.* 2012;185:435–452.
5. Campbell ML, Templin T, Walch J. A Respiratory Distress Observation Scale for patients unable to self-report dyspnea. *J Palliat Med.* 2010;13:285–290.
6. Zernikow B, Michel E, Craig F, Anderson BJ. Pediatric palliative care: use of opioids for the management of pain. *Paediatr Drugs*. 2009;11:129–151.

7. United States Renal Data System (USRDS). 2008 Annual Data Report: Atlas of End-Stage Renal Disease in the United States. National Institutes of Health, National Institute Diabetes and Digestive and Kidney Diseases, 2012. www.usrds.org/adr.htm. Accessed July 7, 2015.
8. Germain MJ, Davison SN, Moss AH. When enough is enough: the nephrologist's responsibility in ordering dialysis treatments. *Am J Kidney Dis*. 2011;58:135–143.
9. Renal Physicians Association. *Shared Decision-Making in the Appropriate Initiation of and Withdrawal From Dialysis: Clinical Practice Guidelines*. 2nd ed. Rockville, MD; Renal Physicians Association; 2010.
10. Jablonski A. Level of symptom relief and the need for palliative care in the hemodialysis population. *J Hospice Palliat Nurs*. 2007;9:50–60.
11. Davison SN, Jhangri GS. Impact of pain and symptom burden on the health-related quality of life of hemodialysis patients. *J Pain Symptom Manage*. 2010;39:477–485.
12. O'Connor NR, Kumar P. Conservative management of end-stage renal disease without dialysis: a systematic review. *J Palliat Med*. 2012;15:228–235.
13. Davison SN, Rosielle DA. Withdrawal of dialysis: decision making #207. *J Palliat Med*. 2012;15:1270–1271.
14. Cohen LM, Poppel DM, Cohn GM, Reiter GS. A very good death: measuring quality of dying in end-stage renal disease. *J Palliat Med*. 2001;4:167–172.
15. Go AS, Mozaffarian D, Roger VL, et al. Executive summary: heart disease and stroke statistics—2013 update. A report from the American Heart Association. *Circulation*. 2013;127:143–152.
16. Grassman D. EOL considerations in defibrillator deactivation. *Am J Hosp Palliat Care*. 2005;22:179; author reply, 180.
17. Park SJ, Milano CA, Tatooles AJ, et al. Outcomes in advanced heart failure patients with left ventricular assist devices for destination therapy. *Circ Heart Fail*. 2012;5:241–248.

Appendix

Self-Assessment Test Questions

Judith A. Paice

Questions

1. When a patient is actively dying, which of the following actions is MOST appropriate?
   A. Monitor vital signs
   B. Insert an indwelling catheter
   C. Position the patient on the left side
   D. Speak quietly and clearly to the patient

2. A family has been told that a patient's comatose condition would probably persist until death. He is still unarousable but is now agitated and extremely restless. The family is uncertain what to do. Which of the following would be the MOST appropriate question to FIRST ask the family?
   A. "When did he last urinate?"
   B. "Does he say anything you can understand?"
   C. "Is there anyone to whom he needs to say goodbye?"
   D. "Has a spiritual advisor been by to see him lately?"
3. A patient has a do-not-resuscitate order. If he is lying on his side, has a respiratory rate of 6 breaths/minute with oropharyngeal congestion, and cold, mottled extremities, the nurse should:
   A. Obtain an order for oxygen
   B. Turn the patient on his back and suction
   C. Administer morphine
   D. Remain available for family support
4. Which of the following is MOST likely occurring when an actively dying patient begins to limit interpersonal involvement?
   A. An expression of anger
   B. A demonstration of depression
   C. An attempt to conserve time and energy
   D. An indirect request for support and attention

5. A patient whose death is imminent is experiencing periods of apnea in between deep and shallow breaths. This describes:
   A. Ataxic breathing
   B. Paradoxical breathing
   C. Cheyne-Stokes breathing
   D. Kussmaul-Kien respirations
6. Which of the following is MOST appropriate for relief of terminal breathlessness?
   A. Oxygen
   B. Opioid
   C. Use of a fan
   D. Semi-Fowler's position
7. A patient with a glioblastoma is actively dying. He begins to exhibit hallucinations and agitation. Which of the following medication should be considered?
   A. Lorazepam
   B. Amitriptyline
   C. Haloperidol
   D. Phenytoin

Answers

1. D
2. A
3. D
4. C
5. C
6. B
7. C

Index

Page numbers followed by *t* or *b* indicate tables or boxes, respectively.